ADOPTION: CHANGING
FAMILIES, CHANGING TIMES

Adoption: changing families, changing times draws together contributions from all those with an interest in adoption: adopted people; birth parents and adoptive parents; practitioners and managers in the statutory and voluntary sectors; academics and policy makers. Chapters on research and policy are interspersed with those from people with first-hand experience of being adopted, becoming an adoptive parent or giving up a child for adoption. Together, they provide unique insights into a subject that although regularly in the media is often surrounded by prejudice and misconception. The editors offer introductions to each section on the context of the issues and debates. Topics covered include:

- children and young people in care
- trying to adopt
- waiting for adoption
- life after adoption
- the politics of adoption.

This accessible text offers a comprehensive review of adoption policy, practice and services and analyses why adoption has become so controversial. It provides professional and general reader alike with a fully rounded picture of adoption and exposes some of the myths surrounding it.

Anthony Douglas is director of social care and health at Suffolk County Council and vice chair of BAAF Adoption and Fostering. **Terry Philpot** is a writer, researcher and journalist on social policy and was formerly editor of *Community Care*.

ADOPTION: CHANGING FAMILIES, CHANGING TIMES

Edited by
Anthony Douglas and
Terry Philpot

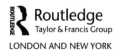

Routledge
Taylor & Francis Group

LONDON AND NEW YORK

First published 2003
by Routledge
11 New Fetter Lane, London EC4P 4EE

Simultaneously published in the USA and Canada
by Routledge
29 West 35th Street, New York, NY 10001

Routledge is an imprint of the Taylor & Francis Group

© 2003 Anthony Douglas and Terry Philpot

Typeset in Sabon by
Florence Production Ltd, Stoodleigh, Devon
Printed and bound in Great Britain by
The Cromwell Press, Trowbridge, Wiltshire

British Library Cataloguing in Publication Data
A catalogue record for this book is available from the British Library

Library of Congress Cataloging in Publication Data
Adoption: changing families, changing times/edited by
   Anthony Douglas and Terry Philpot.
     p. cm.
   1. Adoption – Great Britain. 2. Adoptees – Great Britain.
   3. Adoptive parents – Great Britain. 4. Birthparents – Great Britain.
   I. Douglas, Anthony, 1949– II. Philpot, Terry.
   HV875.58.G7 A32 2003
   362.73′4′0941–dc21   2002068178

ISBN 0–415–25684–4 (hbk)
ISBN 0–415–25685–2 (pbk)

CONTENTS

CONTENTS

CONTENTS

CONTRIBUTORS

Julia Austin is 19 and is studying acting. She lives in London.

Mary Austin grew up in Birmingham and moved to London to start a teaching career with her husband, an educational psychologist. Ten years on, after inconclusive infertility investigations and approaches to adoption agencies, Mary and Mark gave up their jobs and went to Indonesia with VSO, returning three years later with their adopted daughter, Julia. Their son, Robbie, joined the family a week before he was 6. Both children have just begun their college careers. Mary now works as an education consultant with several inner London local education authorities.

Audrey Boundy relinquished her baby son when she was eighteen years old. Twenty-seven years later, he traced her. By then, she was married with a son and daughter, Aline. Audrey is now widowed and still living in Northumberland. **Aline Boundy** is bringing up three young children on her own in Athens, where she teaches. Twenty-four years after contact was made, they are all still in touch.

Felicity Collier has been chief executive of BAAF Agencies for Adoption and Fostering since August 1995. She qualified in social work in 1978 and was awarded an MPhil in social work in 1994. She has previously worked in child care social work, family court welfare and the probation service as practitioner, training manager and assistant chief officer. She wrote the Action Plan for Improving Adoption Services, launched in 1998, much of which has now been acted upon by the government.

Terry Connor has been director, Catholic Children's Society (Arundel and Brighton, Portsmouth and Southwark) since 1982. Previously he worked in London social services departments. He is a trustee and former vice-chairperson of the National Council for Voluntary Child Care Organisations and from 1990 to 1996 was chairperson of British Agencies for Adoption and Fostering. He is currently chair of Caritas in England and Wales. He holds degrees in Spanish and South American Studies.

He is a book reviewer for *Community Care* and most recently published chapters in *The Changing Face of Child Care* (NCVCCO, 2000) and *Authority and Governance in the Roman Catholic Church* (SPCK, 2000).

Joanna Corbett is a professionally qualified and experienced independent social worker who has been employed by and worked for local authorities, and private adoption and fostering agencies placing 'hard to place' children in substitute families since 1983. In 2000 she participated in the production of the BBC TV Programme 'Love is Not Enough' which focused on the process of adoption from the viewpoint of several prospective adoptive families. She is married with two sons and two daughters.

Veronica Dewan is a transracially adopted adult born in 1957. A mental health system survivor, she lives in North London with her partner. Through membership of the Association of Transracially Adopted and Fostered Adults, Veronica has met many young people looking for a safe and supportive place in which to express painful experiences of transracial placement. She is a freelance mental health trainer, consultant and part time MA student in novel and short story writing. She has contributed chapters to anthologies about mental health: *Speaking our minds* (Open University/Macmillan, 1996), and *Something inside so strong* (Mental Health Foundation, 2001).

Anthony Douglas, director of social care and health, Suffolk County Council, is a member of the executive committee of the Association of Directors of Social Services and vice chair of BAAF Adoption and Fostering. He was chair of London ADSS for three years from 1998–2001. He has written two books on British social services: *Caring and coping: a guide to social services* (with Terry Philpot); and *Child protection and adult mental health* (with Amy Weir). He writes regularly for professional journals. He has over twenty years management experience in UK social services, and has held numerous advisory posts in key national policy areas. He is an adoptee.

Julia Feast is manager, post-adoption and care counselling research project, The Children's Society, and, from January 2003, will be policy, research and development consultant, BAAF Adoption and Fostering. She has worked as a local authority social worker and team leader and as a guardian *ad litem* and reporting officer. She is author (with Michael Marwood, Sue Seabrook and Elizabeth Webb) of *Preparing for reunion: experiences from the adoption circle* (The Children's Society, 1994; new edition 2002) and (with David Howe) of *Adoption, search and reunion: the long-term experience of adopted adults* (The Children's Society, 2000). She is also working in the field of the information needs of children born as a result of donor-assisted conception. She is a member of the Department of Health Taskforce on Adoption.

Kirsty Fergusson is a freelance journalist and garden writer. She lives in West Dorset with her four adopted children, three ponies, two dogs and one cat. Before the children, she wrote a PhD on the French philosopher, Michel Tournier, ran a landscape gardening company and for four years was head gardener at Mapperton in Dorset.

Val Forrest has worked for twelve years as a post-adoption counsellor for an adoption team in a London local authority. She is now a senior practitioner with responsibility for assessing prospective adoptive parents, running preparation groups and family finding. She also coordinates a confidential letterbox service, one of the first to be set up by a local authority, with over ninety exchanges a year. She is also a member of an adoption panel. She works freelance for another local authority as a post-adoption counsellor. As part of her MSc in counselling psychology at London University, she carried out research into the support needs of birth mothers.

Jane French lives in London.

Jill Goldson is a senior lecturer and co-ordinator of social work on the Bachelor of Social Practice programme at Unitec, Auckland, New Zealand. Prior to this she has worked extensively with children and families in Britain, Australia and New Zealand. She is currently researching bi-cultural issues for work with vulnerable families.

Gill Gray has fourteen years' experience in children and families social work both at a practitioner and managerial level. She has a special interest in the fields of fostering and adoption. Gill is currently employed as the project leader of the Coram Family Concurrent Planning Project in central London.

Anna Gupta is a lecturer in childcare social work, Royal Holloway College, London University. She is the coordinator of the London Post-Qualifying Child Care Award and also works on the Making Research Count project. She worked for several years as a social worker and team manager with two London boroughs. She has also worked as a guardian *ad litem*. Her main research interests are poverty and race issues in social work with children and families.

Chris Hanvey is UK director of operations, Barnardo's. He has worked with children as both a field worker and in residential care. Until he joined Barnardo's he was chief executive, John Ellerman Foundation, which he joined from the Thomas Coram Foundation (now Coram Family) where he was director. He has also served as director of policy and information, NCH, assistant director of social services, Leeds Council, and principal officer, Coventry social services department. Until last year he was chairperson of an adoption panel for a London borough. He has written extensively on adoption and childcare. He is the author of *Social* *work with mentally handicapped people* (1981) and is co-editor (with Terry Philpot) of *Practising social work* (1994) and *Sweet charity: the role and functions of voluntary organisations* (1996).

Christopher Hignett was born in November 1945. He was adopted and grew up in Leatherhead. He is a senior probation officer working in Inner London and lives with his family in Islington.

Pam Hodgkins has been co-ordinator of the West Midlands Post-Adoption Service since 1994. She was placed for adoption when she was 10 days old and traced both her birth parents in 1982. That year she established the National Organisation for Counselling Adoptees and Parents to assist people involved in the adoption reunion process. She is now a trustee of the organisation. A former teacher in further education, she retrained as a social worker in 1986–8 and was employed as a regional consultant and trainer by British Agencies for Adoption and Fostering. She is a member of the Department of Health's Adoption and Permanence Council and also a member of the Adoption Support Stakeholder Group.

David Howe is professor of social work, University of East Anglia. He has worked as a childcare officer, social worker and team leader before taking up his teaching post at UEA. He has research and writing interests in adoption, attachment theory and child abuse and neglect. He is the author (with Julia Feast) of *Adoption, search and reunion: the long-term experience of adopted adults* (Children's Society, 2000).

Nick Hughes has been a practitioner and manager in children's services for over twenty-two years. He has worked in a range of settings, including youth justice, residential, hospital, fieldwork and family placement. He has worked in both the public and private sectors, and his family placement practice has been undertaken in both shire and metropolitan authorities. Currently he is the service manager for family placements, Sheffield Council.

Karen Irving is chief executive, Parents for Children. Founded in 1976, the agency was the first adoption society in the UK and Europe to help children who had not been thought of for adoption. Karen Irving has twenty-five years' experience in working in fostering and adoption and is chairperson of the Connaught Group of children's charities. She has been awarded a Churchill Memorial Fellowship to undertake further study of methods of helping children who have been maltreated.

Adele Jones is currently a lecturer in social work at the University of the West Indies, St Augustine Campus, Republic of Trinidad and Tobago. Before this, she was a senior lecturer in childcare at Manchester Metropolitan University. She is a qualified social worker, has worked as a local authority family placement officer and is a founder member of the Bibini Centre for Young People in Manchester, an organisation specialising in the care and support of black children and their families. She is also an adoptive parent.

Angela Knight is a freelance writer and producer. Originally a teacher, she then worked for the BBC as a producer in radio then television. In 1989 she moved with her husband to the country after their first daughter, Sasha, was born. After experiencing secondary infertility, an operation to remove a fibroid and three failed traumatic attempts at IVF, Angela turned to adoption. In 1995 she read about babies in overcrowded orphanages in China and went through a two-year adoption process to adopt a seven-month old baby from China. The family is now a foursome, Sasha is twelve years old and Tamzin is five years old – Angela is relieved that IVF failed otherwise they would never have met Tamzin. Angela works as a freelance writer for national newspapers and magazines. She writes children's books, novels and appears on radio and television. One of her aims is to promote adoption and to write and illustrate books about adoption for children who have been adopted.

Donald Macrae was born and educated in Scotland. He studied law at Edinburgh University, and went on to qualify as a lawyer in both England and Scotland. A career civil servant and lawyer, he is currently legal adviser to the Department for Education and Skills.

Sheena Macrae was born in England but brought up and educated in Scotland. Her career as university lecturer and then civil servant was halted by the onset of Crohn's Disease. This caused her infertility and secondary osteoporosis, and ended her career.

Phillip McGill works for a children's charity and was formerly acting manager of a local authority fostering team. He has worked in several different settings in children and families social work services in Scotland and England.

Shelley Mann was born Michelle Evans in 1972. She was taken into foster care by her paternal aunt and uncle when she was nearly two years old. Sixteen years later she was adopted by them. Today she is a graphic designer, living with her partner and young son in Leighton Buzzard, Bedfordshire.

Terry Philpot is a writer on social policy and a regular contributor to several publications including *Times Higher Education Supplement* and *The Tablet*. He was formerly editor of *Community Care*. He has written and edited several books, including *Action for Children*; *Values and Visions: Changing Ideas in Services for People with Learning Difficulties* (with

Linda Ward); *Sweet Charity: The Work and Role of Voluntary Organisations* (with Chris Hanvey); *Caring and Coping: A Guide to Social Services* (with Anthony Douglas); *Political Correctness and Social Work*; and *A Very Private Practice: An Investigation into Private Fostering* (BAAF, 2001). He is currently writing a workbook on adoption, search and reunion for the Children's Society with Julia Feast. He was a member of the Department of Health's Taskforce on Violence against Social Care Staff. He is a trustee of RPS-Rainer and a member of the board of the Social Care Institute for Excellence.

Chris Purnell was born in Leeds in 1945. He left school in 1960 and took exams at night school, followed by a BEd in 1969 and an MA in 1974. He taught for twenty-seven years in East London, and was a councillor in East London between 1990 and 2002. He married in 1969 and has two adult children.

Deborah Savidge and Hugh Maloney met in a crypt, working with the same disaffected group of young people. Hugh runs a housing consultancy project and Debbie is a tutor on a life skills course in London. Their next plan is to take their three children sailing across the Pacific.

John Simmonds is director of policy, research and development at BAAF Adoption and Fostering. Until taking up his present position, he was senior lecturer and programme co-ordinator in social work at Goldsmiths College, University of London. He has had extensive experience in both teaching, research and consultancy in child care practice for over thirty years. He is the father of two adopted children.

June Thoburn is professor of social work, University of East Anglia and is director of the university's Centre for Research on the Child and Family. She has worked as a social worker in England and Canada and has been teaching and researching on a wide range of child welfare topics since 1980. She has particular interests in children and parents and in child placement. She frequently acts as an expert witness in complex child-care and adoption cases. Two of her books are widely read texts: *Child placement: principle and practice* (1994) and (with Clive Sellick) *What works in family placement?* (1996; new edition, with Clive Sellick and Terry Philpot, in press.) Her most recent book (with L. Orford and S. Raschid) is *Permanent family placement for children of minority ethnic origin* (2000).

Penny Thompson has been executive director of social services, Sheffield Council, since 1998. She spent twelve years as a childcare social worker, six of them in Sheffield. She worked as a manager in the former Cleveland County Council before becoming assistant director (children and families), Nottinghamshire County Council. She spent five years as a trustee of British Agencies for Adoption and Fostering, including a period as vice-chairperson. She is currently co-chairperson of the children and families committee of the Association of Directors of Social Services.

Jane Tunstill is professor of social work at Royal Holloway, London University. She has undertaken a wide range of research in the statutory and voluntary child care sectors, including most recently, two consecutive Department of Health funded national studies of the implementation of Section 17 of the Children Act, 1989, and a national study of Family Centres as part of the Department of Health Parenting Initiative. Recent publications include *Making sense of section 17* with Jane Aldgate (HMSO, 1996) and *Children and the state; whose problem?* (Cassell 2000); *Children in need: from policy to practice* (TSO, 2000) She is a member of the National Evaluation of Sure Start research team, with responsibility for the Implementation Study, and a founder member of Making Research Count.

Penelope Welbourne has worked with children and families in a range of social work settings. She is currently a senior lecturer in the Department of Social Work at the University of Plymouth. Her research interests are in the areas of children's rights, and parental stress and child protection.

FOREWORD

There was a time when adoption rarely commanded the attention of newspapers, the public and politicians. A quarter of a century ago the main item of public interest was whether local authorities and voluntary agencies should take up the American idea of advertising children for adoption. Even among professionals at that time the debate about same-race placements was still to get off the ground. The Conservative Government's White Paper, *Adoption – The Future* (Department of Health, 1993) did not get very far past publication and initial discussion. Then professional interest in change was unmatched by political will. There are, though, occasional small hills of attention to observe when looking back on this rather flat landscape of public discourse. And why and how the mood has changed so dramatically to make adoption almost a constant subject of media, public and political interest is both part of the discussion in this book and the book's raison d'être.

Hence the need for what we believe is an unusual and even, we would suggest, a unique book about adoption. It is one that strongly features professional and practice concerns but it is also one that places the whole of its subject within the context not only of public policy but also of the political debate that has informed it. But it is also a book which brings together a wide range of interests and voices, offering differing and different perspectives – not only professionals, academics and practitioners but also birth and adoptive parents, and adopted people; those who have been rejected as adopters and those who have had happy, as well as unhappy adoptions. We cannot fully understand adoption – its importance, its professional and public interest – without taking account of and hearing all those who are party to it. To give some shape to the different issues, the varying aspects and the sometimes contrasting viewpoints, we have divided the contributions into sections and have written our own introductions to offer context.

Given the diversity of social work law and practice even in a small country like the UK – the more so with the coming of devolution – it is wise to mention that almost all references in this book are to English legislation and development (which for our purposes is effectively law for England and Wales). Even the legal recognition of adoption took place at different times in the four countries which make up the UK and the rate of change is sometimes different. For example, as the Adoption and Children Act, which covers England and Wales, was proceeding toward Royal Assent, the review of adoption by the Scottish Executive was still under way. We have included a chapter on New Zealand and there are references in the book to countries overseas, most notably by June Thoburn in her chapter, as well as by those contributors who write about adoption of children from other countries. However, to attempt to cover each country of the UK separately would have made the book cumbersome and to qualify each reference to adoption with a statement that it applied only to England and Wales (where it did) would have made it tedious. We ask our readers' indulgence.

It is our intention, too, that this book should not only be of interest to professionals and those directly concerned with adoption but also to a wider audience. Adoption is tricky: this is all too apparent from some of our contributors. Equally, even for those families where adoption seems to cause no problems, it is a demanding task. In some countries, as is noted, adoption is culturally unacceptable or takes a very different shape from what it does in the UK, the qualifying paragraph above notwithstanding. This needs to be explored and understood. Too much adoption policy is shaped by ignorance at worst and misunderstanding at best. The reforms that have now been enacted by the present government were necessary but they have not always been well informed either in ministerial comment, parliamentary debate or by those who have sought to influence the legislation. We hope that this book goes some way to clarifying and explaining the issues through the words of those who best know the difficulties and satisfactions of seeking to give a child a better life.

Anthony Douglas, Suffolk
Terry Philpot, Surrey
March 2002

INTRODUCTION

It is not so long ago that adoption was seen as an unproblematic solution to the problems facing some children. They came from 'bad' homes or were orphaned or abandoned. Thus, went the argument, as love healed, restored and repaired loss, if such children could only be matched with 'good' families, all would be well. In fact, so potent was the idea that unsatisfactory pasts and even memories could be wiped out, that some of the children were not told they were adopted. Indeed, adopted children were often referred to as 'special' or 'chosen', to distinguish them from other children.

But matters were never really so straightforward and are even less so today. Politicians and the media sometimes present adoption as a simple matter of matching the right (loving) adoptive parents with the right (needy) child. While most adoptions work well, no adoption is simple.

Nearly all of us know someone who is either adopted, adopting or trying to adopt. One in three people are touched by it, directly or indirectly. Eight hundred thousand people in the UK have been adopted and it is reckoned that there are several million others who are affected by adoption – adoptive parents, siblings and other family members, as well as birth parents and birth relatives. Adoption is 'a subject about which most people have information' (Triseliotis et al., 1997).

While adoption became legal in England and Wales only as recently as 1926, it is still very much an Anglo-Saxon institution – a fact which British policy makers sometimes lose sight of. In some European countries (as June Thoburn tells us in chapter 5) there is virtually no adoption. In the US 14 per cent of adoptions are by relatives, whereas most adopters in Britain are people previously unknown to the child. Adoption policy mirrors geopolitics. Britain is not as individualistic as the US, but care is less institutionalised than much of Europe.

The statistics and technical facts of adoption are easy to recount. In the year ending March 2001, 3,420 children were adopted in England. This compares with the 3,125 adopted in the year ending March 2000, 2,880 in 1999 and 2,410 in 1998 (Department of Health, 2001). Three out of four children are adopted from care; the remainder are step-parent adoptions.

1

Adoption follows a court order, which permanently removes all birth parent responsibilities for a child, and transfers full legal rights and responsibilities to an adoptive parent or parents. A child should only be adopted after every effort has been made to protect the child's most precious right – to live happily and safely with its own parent or parents.

We now recognise that adoption can no longer be seen as a surgical break with the birth family and the past. Adopted children have histories which they are entitled to know, and which, in some cases, possibly with professional help, they need to come to terms with. We no longer imagine that being able to adopt the child you have always wanted is without difficulties, or that giving up a child for adoption ends any entitlement of the birth parent to future involvement. Open adoptions, in which contact between the birth parent and child, or between siblings placed with different carers, continues throughout an adoption, are on the increase but still fairly rare. More often than not, they remain fraught emotionally and practically.

Three hundred years ago in the UK, babies were abandoned or murdered if they were unwanted. Indeed, they still are in many countries like China. Adoption was rarely heard of in Britain, although the healthy babies of some poor mothers were sold to wealthy childless couples. Legalisation in England and Wales came seventy-five years after the first laws in America in 1851. American society was built upon displaced children and families coming together to start new lives. Britain, on the other hand, was late in accepting there were alternatives to strong blood ties, and even the first Adoption Act in 1926 which covered England and Wales, did not allow adopted children to inherit from their new parents.

Adoption in some shape or form has taken place in every human society and culture. In ancient Athens, adoption, particularly of boys who were trained to perform religious ceremonies, flourished as early as the fourth century AD. Until adoption became legal, private arrangements were normal, organised by a rogue's gallery of intermediaries. Just as it has been throughout history, the majority of birth parents giving their children up for adoption are unmarried and not in paid work, whereas 95 per cent of adopters are likely to be married, middle class couples with at least one income from a permanent job, and more often than not two.

While trafficking in babies no longer takes place within the UK, it continues as a thriving trade internationally. Thousands of Nepalese girls are trafficked every year into India as child prostitutes. When Nadezdha Fratti, a Russian/Italian was arrested in Volgograd, Southern Russia in 2000, she was suspected of having arranged the illegal adoption in Italy of up to 600 children, mostly babies, during the 1990s. She was paid about £1,700 per child. Fratti is one of many international profiteers who operate as lawyers or adoption brokers. Buyer-led private adoptions are common in the United States, where adoption is comparatively unregulated. In the UK, adopting from abroad can be expensive, with costs ranging from £2,000 for an independent study of suitability, to a five-figure sum if litigation is involved. The infamous Kilshaws, who lost a legal battle to adopt twin baby girls from the US in the first major so-called internet adoption case, had their house in North Wales repossessed after running up legal bills of over £60,000 (*Guardian*, 23 October 2001). A commodification of adoption takes place where bargain-hunting private purchasers with a 'name your price' attitude come into contact with poor families, usually poor mothers, who are tempted by the money they can make, even if they exchange short-term income for long-term sadness at the loss of their baby. Scandals happen in the West too. In the 1940s and 1950s, the Tennessee Children's Home Society in Memphis, US, arranged the illegal adoption for personal profit of at least 1,500 children, in a black market operation orchestrated by its Director, Georgia Tann (Tollet Austin, 1993). Until the Kilshaw case in the UK forced the UK government to make bringing children into the UK without following the correct assessment and approval procedures a criminal offence (Sections 9 and 14 of the Adoption (Intercountry Aspects) Act, 1999), many children in the UK today arrived via this route, and are now growing up adopted all over the country, many of them with little chance of ever finding out the truth about their background. Many, anyway, will have come from countries where records are not available either because they are not advanced bureaucratic states or the ravages of war and civil conflict have destroyed them. Birth, marriage and death records in the Irish Republic went up in flames in 1921 during the siege of the Four Courts in Dublin.

Adopting from abroad is not a contemporary phenomenon, as an excerpt from the leading adoption journal of the time in 1972 shows: 'The Adoption Resource Exchange, for the first time this year found itself with a waiting list of adopters wanting to take a child regardless of colour or race. Seventy-four children found homes in 1971 through the ARE, fifty-two of them fully or partly Negro, the rest Asian' (*Child Adoption*, 1972, vol. 3). What is slightly surprising is that this interest by white families in adopting black children came only three years after the peak year in the UK for the adoption of children by non-related parents, when, in 1968, 16,000 adoption orders were granted in England and Wales, three-quarters being for babies aged one year and under. Just as adoptions within countries still transfer the children of poor parents to richer parents, the same shift takes place between countries. In Russia in 1999, there were only 7,000 domestic adoptions, a declining number, whilst there were equal numbers of foreign adoptions in the same year, two-thirds of the children going to the US. Within the UK, more than 10,000 unaccompanied children are living with friends, relatives or strangers, having made their way here or having been sent from abroad (Kidane, 2001; Philpot, 2001). Some will end up in de facto adoptions. Many, like fifteen-year-old Aslem, who arrived in the UK alone from Afghanistan, miss their homeland: 'I did not choose to come here. I was sent because of the war. I would not choose this for anyone' (BAAF Adoption and Fostering press release, 15 November 2001).

The history of adoption has its ugly side in every single country. As a result of investigations into stolen Aboriginal children in Australia, who were taken from their families and placed in church-run missions to rescue them from, or cure them of their aboriginality, child care policy in Australia today is that Aboriginal children being placed in substitute care should be placed within their own culture and community. The *Daily Mail* airlifted over 100 children out of Vietnam at the end of the Vietnam War and brought them to England. Many spent their childhood not happily adopted, but in residential care in the UK. Rescuing as an act of mercy often leads to worse consequences than those originally faced. Above all, many of the children forcibly removed from their homes or homelands dream of either going back or re-establishing contact. One of the Vietnamese children, Minh Le, now in his thirties, carries around a faded photograph of the sister he left behind in Saigon, who he will never see again (*Guardian*, 6 August 2001). Many countries, like Romania and China, which had no child care services of note a decade ago, are now developing family placement services of their own, to the extent that Romania now bans foreign adoptions.

Despite these risks and tragedies, adoption has generally been a successful social policy. Numerous studies over the last 50 years have demonstrated that the outcomes for children in care, especially younger children, are better after adoption than in long-term foster care or residential care, although there was not always a consensus about the distinguishing factors. (A selection of studies are listed at the end of this chapter.) As disproportionately more children in care end up homeless, in prison, under psychiatric care, or adrift in the job market without skills and qualifications, it is important to maximise the security and stability a positive adoption can give to children and young people who have suffered a wretched early childhood, which can include being chronically neglected or subjected to long-term physical sexual and emotional abuse. Seventy-five per cent of children in long-term care leave school without a single GCSE grade C or above. Fifty per cent of children who have been in care are jobless a year after leaving care. Thirty-four per cent of homeless young people are care leavers. Twenty-three per cent of the adult prison population have been in the care system. Sixty per cent of male prostitutes have been in care (NCH Action for Children, 2000). A superficial reading of the figures about children in care propelled Prime Minister Blair to see adoption as a cure-all.

While statistics always need to be treated with caution, and cannot be generalised to outcomes for individual children, adoption tends to make children feel more stable and secure in a new family, even in a step family. As a friend of one of the editors (Anthony Douglas) wrote about her stepfather after his death: 'Darling Michael, the biggest truth I have realised in all my life in the last fifty-two years since you adopted me is that you have been the most loving stepfather a child could ever have had' (Nesbitt, 2001). Step-parent adoptions form a constantly diminishing percentage of all UK adoptions, and there is a case for dealing with them administratively in registry offices, rather than judicially. Indeed, when thinking about adoption, it is important to keep in mind the three main types: adopting from care, international adoption and step-family adoption. Their very different characteristics are yet another reason why adoption cannot be seen as straightforward. Nor can those affected be regarded as a homogeneous group.

As one in three marriages in the UK end in divorce, and as many partners either re-marry or find a new long-term relationship outside marriage, step-parent adoption is a way of binding children from a first marriage into a second. Most step-parent adopters are men, but the total number of step-parent adoptions is tiny compared with the number of unmarried partners living together and bringing up children within a stable long-term relationship.

Most adopters who adopt internationally are child-centred couples, contemplating adoption as a third-best option for family-forming, after discovering they cannot produce children of their own, and in many cases after unsuccessful fertility treatment. There are some, too, who have children of their own but decide to add to their family through adoption. It may be that in the future, human cloning will make adoption unnecessary. What would happen then to rejected children? For now, understandably, most couples in this position would prefer to adopt a baby who could be theirs from the word go. Early enquiries soon acquaint would-be adopters with the fact that adoption agencies in the UK, seeking homes for children in the care system, are looking to match children with special needs with parents with special talents. Children will often be older, they may well have a serious disability, or they may be part of a complicated sibling group. Indeed, one of the facts which has altered adoption out of all recognition in a generation is the paucity of babies now available for adoption: 8,500 in England and Wales in 1970, and in 2000, just 200. As a result, many childless couples decide to adopt a child from abroad.

The third and most complex group of children in the adoption system are children in care. It is their stories that occupy most of our attention as editors of this book. Many of the adopters in our book have adopted children who have waited, or children who have been let down time and time again. Their stories demonstrate both the reality of adoption today, but optimistically, the inescapable conclusion that there are 'parents for children, not children for parents' to be found, if family finders search long, hard and astutely enough (Fowler, 2001).

Many prospective adopters continue to report that adoption agencies, particularly local authorities, cause unnecessary delays, burden them with paper work and generally act in all kinds of ways that feel either deliberately obstructive or indifferent to the urgency they feel, and the urgency those same prospective adopters feel that children waiting to be adopted will be feeling. Some adopters view adopting from abroad as a faster process which fits in better with their life plans. It is undoubtedly the case that many adopters who go overseas would be willing and able to look after children who need adopting from care, if family finding was dealt with through a coordinated national system. The new National Adoption Register will help by building on existing national matching services like the BAAF Adoption and Fostering magazine *Be my parent*, which features individual children needing adoptive homes, and which is available nationally. A cautionary note should be struck. Only 25 per cent of the children referred to *Be my parent* in the last year ended up being adopted. The remainder stayed in long-term foster care placements or returned to their birth families. As we discuss in more detail later in this chapter, the government's new adoption targets are unrealistic, unless twice as many adopters can be found.

Professional practice in adoption is often unfairly criticised by those who do not appreciate or accept that potential adopters need to be rigorously assessed, and it may not be possible to match particular adopters with a child who is waiting. This is like a homeless person seeing an empty home and immediately demanding to live in it, oblivious to the fact that there may be other homeless people who have been waiting longer, in greater need, or that the house itself may need underpinning before anyone can live in it again. Such an attitude seems to be based on the curious overlooking of the fact that adoption is a service for children, not one for people who cannot have their own children or wish to add to their family by adopting. But over the last ten years, a number of adoption agencies have joined forces and set up adoption consortia, pooling the children who need a placement and the adopters who are available to take a child, in order to increase the number of matching options.

Ideally, following an assessment that a child needs a permanent substitute family, the child will be freed for adoption legally, a suitable adopter will be identified and thoroughly prepared, including being given all the available information about the child, and the child will be placed without delay, with the placement receiving a high level of post-placement or post-adoption support. In reality, there is a gulf between theory and practice. The assessment process may not be instantly conclusive, in that it is hard to judge whether poor parenting in the past inevitably means parenting will repeat itself if the child returns home. Parents can change, and many do, especially if they are supported as a family after their child returns home, as eight children out of ten do. There may well be delays in the court process, either because of timetabling problems or the need for court welfare staff to make a succession of time-consuming enquiries before they can be clear what to advise a magistrate or judge. Complex decisions in other fields take years for courts to determine, and the trend to citizenship gives rights to many parties in a process as complex as adoption. Post-adoption support cannot be funded in some parts of the country. When things go wrong for a child in care, it is often for a number of reasons, some relating to resources, some to professional practice. That of course is little consolation for those directly involved. Most children and adopters can live with short-term setbacks. What is unforgivable is a delay in the adoption process stretching on for years, so that all involved lose heart and the adoption breaks down. One of the saddest groups of children in the care system are those who have been in care, who have at long last been adopted and whose adoptions then break down so they end up back in the care system yet again. Adoption breakdown is another fact sidestepped by those who see adoption as a childcare panacea.

Such are some of the facts of adoption. But the comparatively small number of annual adoptions cannot easily explain the disproportionate amount of media, public and political attention which the subject attracts. While Alan Milburn, Secretary of State for Health, has said that too often adoption has been the last resort for children, when it should be the first (Milburn, 2001), he knows little of which he speaks. Even if local authorities – who are the main adoption agencies, despite the work in the voluntary sector – were to improve practice more than they have and resources were not a question, there would never be more than 4–5,000 children available for adoption. The prime minister – perhaps, significantly, the son of an adopted father – early on took the lead in seeing adoption as a solution to the needs of children in care and personally chaired the interdepartmental committee which led to the Adoption and Children Act 2002. Yet there are 58,100 children currently (2002) in the care of local authorities. The overwhelming majority are not, and will never be available for adoption: they are living with their families while subject to a care order, they are in temporary foster homes, they will return to their families or they do not wish to be adopted.

By comparison, consider not merely children who live in poverty or, nearer, in practice and policy terms to adopted children, the 35,000 children who are fostered. The latter get hardly any political, media or public attention at all and the former, while not ignored, get far, far less than their numbers or condition warrant.

No, there are other reasons why adoption commands the attention that it does. True, most adopted people do not consciously think about their situation day to day. For them, for all practical and emotional purposes, their adopted family is their family. Like almost everyone else they get on with their lives, have their achievements and strive to overcome those difficulties which they share with the unadopted majority of the population.

But however much the adopted person goes about his or her life in much the same way as the unadopted neighbour, there are other, deeper currents at play in the public arena than the simple, laudable wish to provide more children with satisfactory homes. It is not, then, just a matter of how adoption affects the adopted person and their birth and adopted families. At its most profound level, adoption touches something deep in the human psyche. For example, many of us who are not adopted commonly fantasise that we are not the children of our parents but the lost or abandoned offspring of more romantic figures.

Adoption intersects with notions of the family. The stories of Moses, Oedipus and many a fairy tale give imaginative expression to our preoccupations about origins and identity. Mike Leigh's 1995 film *Secrets and Lies* deals with what is now a common experience (or at least an almost universal consideration) for adopted people – the search for those who gave them birth. Of the 800,000 adopted people in Britain, it is estimated that 300,000 have actively engaged in such a search.

This human interest in adoption is witnessed frequently elsewhere in our popular culture. Other films like *Stuart Little* (1999) and *Big Daddy* (2000) cover the complexities of adoption through use of humour and a happy ending, especially for children. P. D. James' *Innocent blood* (James, 1980) has a young woman who seeks her adopted mother only to find that she is a murderess. This is a less a thriller making use of the device of adoption as a Jamesian exploration of a now not uncommon human situation. Margaret Forster has written two novels where adoption is at the centre of human drama. The first, *The Battle for Christabel* (Forster, 1990) is less about a struggle to adopt, as its title might suggest, as the struggle between contending parties in an adoption case. Her later work, *Shadow Baby* (Forster, 1996) concerns the search for roots in the stories of two women, born generations apart but whose childish fates tie them together. Dave Pelzer wrote the best selling trilogy, *A child called it*, *The lost boy*, and *A man named Dave*, based upon a young man who was placed in substitute family care after an early childhood dominated by harrowing abuse (Pelzer, 1995, 1997, 1999). Harry Potter is now perhaps the most world's most famous orphan, as well as wizard. Harry's parents were killed by Voldemort – 'he who must not be named' – and Harry was brought up by his cruel aunt and uncle, Mr and Mrs Dursley, who denied him the truth and information about his parents, who he longed for (Rowling, 1997). Harry Potter belongs to a long tradition of children's literature and fairy tales where a child or children are separated from their birth parents and placed in substitute families. Family placement is familiar territory for children's books, like *The story of Tracy Beaker* (Wilson, 1991) and *Dustbin Baby* (Wilson, 2001).

Thus, into this psychological and cultural cauldron we cast the debates that surround public policy. Public policy, the effects of secrecy and a wish to know who we are coincided tragically in the case of the anonymous man who wrote to the *Guardian*:

> My father hated and bullied me, cheated on my mother for years (as she did on him), and gambled and drank us into misery. I left the family as soon as I could, keeping in touch only with my sister. When I was 40, my sister told me what everybody had known but me: he wasn't my father . . . Knowing I have been lied to all my life is unendurable. I can't believe anything about myself any more. I'm not interested in tracing my 'real' family; I just want to know I'm worth

the truth. My motives aren't purely selfish. The illness that forced my retirement from work has appeared in my son, and I am terrified in case it's inherited from my unknown father.

(Guardian, 1 June 2001)

Individual rights is one of the key themes now affecting how social policy and adoption in particular develops. A single adoption is often a battleground between competing rights. Fifty years ago, birth parents had far fewer rights than today, as did relatives like grandparents. Today, the child, one or two birth parents, relatives from the child's extended family, potential adopters and a local authority acting in *loco parentis*, may all have rights but may not all agree on what is in the best interests of a particular child. In many ways it is remarkable that in over 40 per cent of state-sponsored adoptions, all parties involved do end up agreeing. Contested adoptions can be extremely tricky for courts to determine. It is that trickiness that often leads to delays in making a final adoption order, or indeed in reaching a final decision that a child should return home because life there is much improved. The government wishes to speed up the adoption process for children in the care system, but this assumes that competing rights can be assessed, resolved and decided, often judicially, within a few months. Children, of course, should not wait a day longer than is necessary for a permanent home to be found. The reality is also that adoption agencies have staff shortages and their own competing pressures. While the ideal is for every stage in the process to move quickly and smoothly without undue delay, there are no short cuts in adoption work. Rushing into the wrong placement is as catastrophic as a delay in finding the right one. The consequences can be lifelong, either way.

Adoption law reform comes in periodic waves about once every quarter of a century, each time following a movement for change led by key professional and academic figures. 1926, 1948, 1976 and now 2002, are the key dates in the calendar, although, it can be argued that the latest changes came as a result of media and political pressure more than professional energy. Changes consulted about for the Adoption and Children Act, 2002 included proposals to simplify the court process, and to introduce stronger performance measures for local authorities, including a target of increasing adoptions from care by 40–50 per cent in the next three to four years (2001), a target greeted at the outset with incredulity by adoption professionals, especially as the number of care orders made by courts in England rose to 6,299 in the year 2000, from 4,124 in the previous year, an unprecedented leap of 52.7 per cent (Lord Chancellor's Department, 2001).

Whatever satisfactions today's policy makers and agitators in parliament may gain from the new reforms, they are, in many ways, about numbers. This is not to neglect the fact that if the numbers of satisfactory placements rise a greater number of children will be offered the possibility of a better life. However, the decade which saw the most radical, influential and long-lasting reforms was the 1970s. Here adoption came into its own in the UK. Academics like Roy Parker of Bristol University first pressed publicly for permanency planning for children in long-term care, seeking a fundamental shift away from residential care to family care as the main placement option for children in care. Other countries like the US also had their own strong permanency movement around this time. Thirty years later, that vision has come about with over 70 per cent of children in care in the UK now placed with families, either through fostering or adoption, the overwhelming majority with foster carers. Organisations like Parents for Children, whose chief executive Karen Irving has written a contribution to this book, was set up in 1976 by two sets of parents who had themselves adopted children. 'Their radical idea was to bring together the two groups missed by the adoption system: children considered unadoptable, and families turned away because they were too old, single parents or who didn't meet some of the other criteria' (interview in the *Highbury and Islington Express*, 20 April 2001).

It is unfortunate that we do not hear more from successful adopters and happily placed children, although an increasing number of personal stories are appearing on the internet and elsewhere. Rejected adoption applicants get far more air and screen time and column inches. As Martin Amis says:

> We live in the age of mass loquacity. We are all writing it or at any rate talking about it: the memoir, the apologia, the CV, the *cri de coeur*. Nothing, for now, can compete with experience … We are surrounded by special cases, by special pleadings, in an atmosphere of universal celebrity … It's not the case that in the future everyone will be famous for fifteen minutes. In the future, everyone will be famous all the time – but only in their own minds.
>
> (Amis, 2000)

We live in an age of self-revelation, angst and emotional chaos. Newspaper columns are full of individual's life stories condensed into a few hundred words, many of them famous. The comedian Jim Davidson has talked widely about his adoption, and his search for identity through various marriages, always searching for the right woman – his mother? At least one of those relationships was alleged to have been violent, perhaps as each adult relationship failed to match up to his impossible expectations (*Sunday People*, 21 October 2001). John Lennon employed private detectives and used the media extensively in a search for his sister, who was relinquished for adoption at birth. They never met (Mullender, 1999). Bill Clinton and Marilyn Monroe were adopted. Louis Emerick, who plays Mick Johnson in the long running Channel 4 soap 'Brookside', and who was also adopted, said:

> I only discovered I was adopted when I was 11. I had always assumed that I had come out of my mother's womb. I tortured myself as to

why my mother gave me away as a baby. I traced my birth mother and met her at Lime Street Station in Liverpool. I grew to understand why she gave me away. She was a single mother with a mixed race baby. In the 1950s, that just wasn't accepted. I would have been brought up in a predominantly white area of Merseyside – and who knows how tough that might have been. I wouldn't have been the person I am now, with a father whom I worship – who is now my hero. She thought she was doing the right thing, and in retrospect, I think she did.

(Hello magazine, 2 October 2001)

All adoptions, however happy, leave a residue of confusion and doubt. The most important issue is to understand your past and to come to terms with it. But it is just these personal stories and, most of all, those of people who have been rejected as adoptive parents, which have fuelled the belief that social services departments are infected by political correctness, that they allow children to languish, unnecessarily, in care, and that they give adoption a low priority. In short, such stories, retailed by newspapers and politicians, have given credence to the idea that adoption is a simple matter of finding the right child for the right family – and, as so many couples have been (allegedly) unfairly rejected, that far, far more children could be rescued from care.

Conservative commentators like Patricia Morgan contend 'that political correctness drives current adoption practice; that prospective adopters are disqualified for spurious reasons; that social workers are dogmatic about transracial adoption; and that inadequate parenting of the poor is tolerated because of a misguided cocktail of parental rights and family preservation policies' (Connor, 1998). Commentators from the opposite end of the political spectrum contend that transracial placements are nearly always bad for children, even in the absence of a viable same race alternative. Black issues have remained an uneasy and unresolved undercurrent of adoption policy and practice in the UK for the last twenty-five years, with practitioners often taking an opposite and less populist point of view to politicians. This, in turn, has left adoption social workers and managers trapped in the middle of a stark and often uncompromising debate. Black children in care have clearly benefited over the last twenty years by the greater availability of same race placements, especially as racism in many UK communities shows no sign of easing, even if the form it takes and those it involves changes.

Adoption seems to affect politicians more powerfully than most social issues, on a personal level. British Prime Ministers like John Major and Tony Blair have taken up the cudgel, often through personally knowing disaffected potential adopters who were turned down by local authorities or who were trying to adopt from overseas and who felt they were subject to a form of character assassination by social workers. Politicians and the media continue to promote illiberal adoption politics, which usually consists of praising inter-country adopters and haranguing gays and lesbians who might wish to adopt. Any social worker will tell you that some children, like girls who have been sexually abused by their fathers or male partners of their mothers, prefer a same sex placement. Myth and reality are often wildly unrelated when adoption is politicised, nowhere more strongly than in reactions to gay and lesbian adoption (Holloway, 2002).

Adoption law and policy moves in a conservative way, compared to the wider social changes in family life over the last half century. This book seeks to describe adoption from the perspectives of the key participants in the process: people who have been adopted, practitioners, birth parents, those who have adopted, managers of services and others. Our contributors speak with unique and often powerful voices, frequently borne out of deep experience. Like them, as editors, we offer insights – not all of which coincide – rather than solutions to the dilemmas adoption today poses. We hope we have managed to convey both the benefits and the drawbacks of adoption to a general readership as well as to those already playing a part in the adoption community in one role or another.

References

Amis, M. (2000), *Experience*, London, Jonathan Cape.

Connor, T. (1998) Review of *Adoption and the care of children*, (Morgan, P., IEA, London), *Community Care*, 19 November.

Department of Health (2001), *Social services statistics: children adopted from care in year ending 31 March 2001*, London, Department of Health.

Forster, M. (1990), *The battle for Christabel*, Harmondsworth, Penguin Books.

Forster, M. (1996), *Shadow baby*, London, Chatto and Windus.

Fowler, A. (2001), *Stories of adoption*, London, Parents for Children.

Holloway, Dr J. (2002), *Homosexual parenting: does it make a difference? A re-evaluation of the research with adoption and fostering in mind*, Newcastle East Paediatric Team.

James, P. D. (1980), *Innocent blood*, London, Faber & Faber.

Kidane, S. (2001), *Food, shelter and half a chance*, London, BAAF Adoption and Fostering.

Lord Chancellor's Department (2001), *Industrial statistics*, London.

Milburn, A. (2001), Second Reading of the Adoption and Children Act, 29 October. London, Hansard.

Mullender, A. (ed.) (1999), *We are family: sibling relationships in permanent family placement and beyond*, London, British Agencies for Adoption and Fostering.

NCH Action for Children (2000), *Factfile 1999: facts and figures on issues facing Britain's children*, London, NCH Action for Children.

Nesbitt, G. (2001), *Michael*, Wytherston Farm, Powerstock, Bridport, Dorset.

Pelzer, D. (1995, 1997, 1999), *A child called it; The lost boy; A man named Dave*, London, Orion Books.

Philpot, T. (2001), *A very private practice: an investigation into private fostering*. London, BAAF Adoption and Fostering.

Rowling, J. K. (1997), *Harry Potter and the philosopher's stone*, London, Bloomsbury.

Tollet Austin, L. (1993), *Babies for sale*, Connecticut, Praeger Publishers.

Triseliotis, J., Shireman J. and Hundleby M. (1997), *Adoption: theory, policy and practice*, London, Cassell.

Wilson, J. (1991), *The story of Tracy Beaker*, London, Doubleday Books.

Wilson, J. (2001), *Dustbin baby*, London, Doubleday Books.

Selected studies on the outcomes of adoption

Sophie Van. S. Theis (1924), *How foster children turn out*, New York, State Charities Aid Association.

Skodak, M. and Skeels, H. M. (1949), A final follow up study of 100 adopted children, *Journal of Genetic Psychology*, 75, pp. 85–125.

Witmer, H. L., Herzog, E., Weinstein, E. A. and Sullivan, M. E. (1963), *Independent adoptions*, New York, Russell Sage Foundation.

McWhinnie, A. M. (1967), *Adopted children – how they grow up: a study of their adjustment as adults*, London, Routledge.

Kornitzer, Margaret (1968), *Adoption and family life*, London, Putnam.

Tizard, Barbara (1977), *Adoption: a second chance*, London, Open Books.

Raynor, Lois (1980), *The adopted child comes of age*, London, George Allen & Unwin.

Part I

CHILDREN AND YOUNG PEOPLE IN CARE

INTRODUCTION

Of the 60,000 children in care in the UK, the vast majority will go home to their families. A quarter of these will be over the age of 16. Only 15 per cent are aged between 0 and 4 years. Most of these children will also go back home to their families. There are between 4,000 and 5,000 adoptions in total each year, which includes private law adoptions like step-parent adoptions. 3,067 children, slightly more than half the total, were adopted from care during 2000–01, of whom only 200 were babies. This was 12 per cent more as a total than in the previous year, and over 40 per cent more than in 1998–9 (Department of Health statistics). A further 1,000–2,000 children in the care system could and should be adopted from care annually. On average a child in local authority care can expect to wait a little under three years before being placed with an adoptive family. These figures vary enormously between local authorities, for a number of reasons. In some councils, 10 per cent of children looked after are adopted, whereas in others the figure is less than 2 per cent, but often like is not being compared with like. Adoptions are often like buses; in some months you get none at all because of circumstances, then several come in a rush. And sometimes, for perfectly good reasons, adoption isn't what's needed for children in a local care system.

Being brought up in a substitute family has inevitable and frequently complex repercussions for personal identity. David Blagdon, a career criminal with convictions for arson and blackmail, received a life sentence at Oxford Crown Court in 1978 for setting fire to the curtains at a church in South Hinksey after the death of both his foster parents within days of each other. He was released in 2002 after a campaign by friends and relatives. 'Changes of carer in the first year of life can cause damage to an infant's early brain development. An early placement, preferably in the first few weeks, enables a child's attachment and trust in adults to take root and grow. Multiple placements lead to a "superficial promiscuous personality". After multiple moves, the child despairs and ceases to trust' (Cameron, 2000). Even when a child achieves stability, as Blagdon did, it is too late. Hereditary illness, often thought to be a major risk factor in adoptions, is far less significant than current behaviour caused by situational and environmental factors. Whereas it is estimated that 18 per cent of adopted children have a hereditary risk factor of some description, 40 per cent of adopted children have a level of developmental delay (Ivaldi, 2000a).

Attachment is the key issue, not adoption. The right long-term placement for a child in care is usually the one which ensures a lasting unbroken attachment, based upon re-parenting. Attachment deficits show up time and time again as one of the key environmental factors driving serious anti-social acts like homicides committed by people with mental health problems, as evidenced in inquiry reports. Without a decent attachment, adults will often search hopelessly and unsuccessfully for a caring parent for the whole of their adult lives, starting and ending catastrophic serial relationships. However, what is true for one child, or adult for that matter, does not hold for another. As Penelope Welbourne shows in her contribution, older children can often survive damaging early experience and do well in a late adoption. One of the editors will never forget working with a 17-year-old in care, who only came into care aged 15, who desperately wanted to be adopted by his foster carers before his eighteenth birthday. 'We made it by a few days!!'

Attachment is an equal issue for adopters. To bond with a child who isn't your own is a complicated developmental process, however much adopters have yearned for a child. Sometimes, adopters realise they have made a mistake and pull out in time. At other times, it is one parent who is the driving force, and the other never properly bonds, as indeed can happen with birth parents. Assessing the quality of a relationship between potential adopters, their staying power over a couple of decades when their own circumstances change, and their skills at nurturing insecure and often damaged children, can only ever be an approximate art. Success rates are high, although when an adoption goes wrong, it can have fatal consequences. John Anthony Smith was 4 years old when he was killed by his prospective adoptive parents, Simon and Michelle McWilliam, in Brighton, on Christmas Eve in 1999. When he died, he had fifty-four bruises and four bite marks on his body. His hair had been torn out. The McWilliams were jailed for 8 years in October 2001. They were a manipulative couple who deceived social workers throughout the assessment process about their backgrounds. Mr McWilliam's previous two wives would have disclosed domestic violence – he had changed his name twice – and Mrs McWilliam had five criminal convictions. Too great a reliance was placed on the account the prospective adopters gave of their background, and not enough on checks from other, independent sources (Brighton and Hove Area Child Protection Committee, 2001). This is a salutary case to bear in mind when applicants complain about the intrusiveness of the assessment process for becoming an adopter. Adopters do sometimes adopt for lifestyle reasons – Faith Popcorn, the American trend forecaster who set up BrainReserve, says of her adopted daughter G.G., who she adopted from China at the age of 50, 'You don't expect a woman of my age to have a 2½-year-old child. It has allowed people to see me in a more human way' . . . to which a reporter said, 'Popcorn has used her kid to reposition herself' (*Sunday Times* magazine, December 2000).

Legally, an adoption can be formalised when a baby is 6 weeks old. Parents, usually a single mother where babies are concerned, have 6 weeks to decide whether or not to keep their baby, even if they have previously decided not to. Calls to shorten this to 48 hours fail to recognise the time it takes a mother to think straight in the first few days and weeks after giving birth. These days, relinquishing or abandoning a baby is rare, partly because parenting conveys an entitlement to state housing and benefits, albeit with far less generous provision than in many other Western European countries, and partly because attitudes to teenage pregnancy and lone parenthood are less condemning than they were a generation ago. If anything, we have gone too far the other way, as we now have one of the highest rates of teenage pregnancy in Europe. At the same time, the average age a woman has her first child is rising, and children are leaving home much later. Social trends are changing rapidly. The fastest growing category of new householders is single people over 30 years old. As far as adoption goes, these trends all contribute to the reduction in the number of babies available for adoption, and the number of young couples eager to adopt. Of the 200 babies or so adopted every year, black infants under 6 months old wait on average 10 months for a placement, compared to 3 months for white infants and 4 months for those of mixed ethnicity. These discrepancies carry on for older children in relation to adoption. Black and ethnic minority children are more likely to be the subject of a plan for long term fostering than white children, and white children are more likely to be placed for adoption. And even in long-term fostering, black and ethnic minority children wait longer than white children (BAAF, 2000b; Ivaldi, 2000a). Institutional racism is endemic in the family placement system.

The younger the child in care, the more likely their care plan will be for adoption. In a study of 220 children in local authority care, Lowe *et al.* found that the mean age of children for whom adoption was the care plan was 5.5 years, as opposed to 9.6 years where the plan was for long-term fostering. Of the children for whom adoption was the plan, 64 per cent were aged 1–4 years, 25 per cent aged 5–9 years and 11 per cent 10–12 years. One year later, 19 per cent of the children had experienced a change of plan, whilst only 7 per cent of the total sample in the study had been adopted. Three per cent of placements had broken down – four children in long-term foster care placements and two in adoptive placements (Lowe *et al.*, 2001). The findings confirm the reality of day-to-day child care practice in local authorities and other adoption agencies. Circumstances in the lives of children and families change frequently, and plans have to follow suit. Placing children for adoption, especially older children, is a long complicated and risky business. Worryingly, Lowe *et al.* found that only 61 per cent of children for whom adoption was the care plan had clear reasons for the plan recorded. It is likely that with greater clarity about care planning, as well as better support for adopters before and after placement, the success rate for adoptions would dramatically increase (Lowe *et al.*, 2001). Many children have not been well served by local authorities, who raised their expectations they would make the future better for them. In the 1980s, for example, children were often prepared for adoption, even though no-one was ever found. Children clung onto their life story books, which were photographic portraits of their lives to date, longing for a new mummy and daddy. Many ended up with neither their old ones nor a new one. Those children who do move have often had to move several times in their lives already, involving loss of friends, loss of school and as many would see it, compulsory removal from familiar surroundings.

Preparing a child to be adopted is a complex process, for which there are few short cuts. A range of excellent storybooks have been written which explains each step of the adoption process to children – *Hoping for the Best* (Byrne and Chambers, 1997), *Joining Together* (Byrne and Chambers 1998), and *Waiting for the Right Home* (Byrne and Chambers, 2001); *Chester and Daisy Move On* – a story about two bear cubs who are adopted (Lidster, 1995); and *Nutmeg Gets Adopted* (Foxon, 2001). Matching a baby or very young child is usually a process of selecting good adopters, who would be capable of looking after any child of the preferred age. Matching older children is a different process, which also includes finding out from children what they want or need. Older children often have brothers and sisters they may or may not want to be placed with, they will have views about whether or not they are advertised in journals, and they will wish to express views about any potential adopters selected for them before they are placed. Children and young people frequently attend adoption panels where decisions are being taken about them, and express strong views directly to decision makers, which often contradict professional opinion.

Forty per cent of children in the care system have special needs like a learning disability, a physical disability or medical problems. In most European countries, they would remain in residential care rather than be adopted. Caring for a seriously disabled child is tough. It requires 24-hour care, and can quickly become life-threatening if medication regimes are not complied with. Residential care is much easier. Staff work in shifts and often in pairs. Some children need two or even three staff to care for them, such is the combination of their physical needs and challenging behaviour. That is why it is remarkable that in the UK so many disabled children are looked after in families with foster carers and adopters. It is a real national achievement. The stories of profoundly disabled children who have been adopted are powerful and inspirational (Argent, 1998). They will have additional concerns over and above non-disabled children in care, such as 'Do they know I can't walk? Are they strong enough to lift me? Will my wheelchair go in? Will they understand me when I talk funny? Will they give me my injections?

Will they stay with me in hospital?' The ultimate question all children in care, disabled or non-disabled, fret about is, 'what happens if they can't manage?' (Argent and Kerrane, 1997).

A BAAF study on the work of voluntary adoption agencies looked at 944 children referred for adoption to the agencies by local authorities in the four years to 1998 (Ivaldi, 2000b). Of these, 63 per cent were said to have emotional difficulties, and 46 per cent had behavioural problems. This is why social workers often seek adopters who have either brought up their own children or had considerable experience of caring for children in a professional capacity like teaching. Children in need can behave in ways which test out even the greatest desire to parent a child. As the well-researched BBC series on 'Adoption, Love Is Not Enough', concluded, love is essential, but other personal qualities and most of all, parenting skills, are just as important (BBC, 2000).

Frank Kunstal identifies seven qualities of therapeutic parents, which set out the strengths parents who adopt older children or children with special needs require (Kunstal, 1998):

1   A style of thinking beyond behaviour and into the child's needs, feelings and dilemmas.
2   A capacity to develop a 'caring' connection to the child.
3   A focus on education and correction rather than punishment, in response to misbehaviour.
4   A recognition of and openness to change ineffective reactions to the child's misbehaviour.
5   An emotional acceptance of the child's past and an appreciation of tenuous connections.
6   A commitment to caring and refusal to be rejected.
7   A belief that healing will occur, an appreciation of small gains, and the patience to press for change as a 'test of time'.

The 1998–9 National Adoption Survey, of UK local authorities, showed that children adopted from care in 1999 were much younger than in 1994, at 4 years 3 months on average compared with 5 years 10 months in 1994. 25 per cent of children were placed with their adopters under the age of 1 compared with only 20 per cent over 5. Children also spent a shorter time in care prior to being adopted – 3 years 1 month in 1999, compared with 3 years 8 months in 1996 (BAAF, 2000a). This recent improvement in performance, coupled with new National Standards for Adoption launched by the Department of Health in August 2001, gives grounds for cautious optimism that the needs of children in the care system who cannot return home are being addressed with a greater degree of urgency.

Concurrent planning, also known as dual planning, dual tracking or parallel planning, recognises the fact that it is not always clear when a child comes into care whether the child will be able to go back home or whether they may need long-term care with foster carers or adoptive carers. Concurrent planning means that the child care plan allows two plans to be developed in tandem, one for a return home, the other a contingency plan for a fostering or adoptive placement, with carers who would be happy to either foster or adopt, depending on how the situation develops. Sequential planning can easily take up to three years for an individual child, which is far too long to leave most children in limbo. Several American states have included concurrent planning explicitly in their child care legal framework. Gill Gray discusses concurrent planning in depth in Chapter 3.

Kinship care by relatives achieves less prominence in Britain than in many countries, including the US. As Broad *et al.* found, 'there are major organisational and funding problems which discourage kinship care ... the disadvantages of kinship care centre on two main themes, so far as young people and carers were concerned. These were the limits it placed on their own lifestyle (especially the carers) and the financial hardship both young people and carers suffer. Emotional conflict with other family members was a disadvantage for many carers (Broad *et al.*, 2001). Another common theme that relatives like grandparents express is that they could do more if they had better financial and practical help before and after placement from social services.

In the developed countries, relationships are the war zones of our age. Children who are brought here to be adopted from real war zones, often find themselves at some stage in their childhood witnessing family breakdown or serious tensions. That is the reality in the lottery of long-term relationships, all of which start out aiming to be successful, but many of which do not make it. Many adopted children who have been in care do not expect things to work out:

> Joyce, like most children, wanted to be adopted, liked her adoptive parents, and was upset when the adoption disrupted. For a very few children, however, a disrupted adoption is not a tragic event but a familiar happening. Leaving a family is something they know and are comfortable with: the idea of permanence, an unknown entity, is too frightening. Some children manipulate their own rejection, in order to terminate the adoption. Much more work needs to be done with these children in preparing them for re-placement.
>
> (Fitzgerald, 1983)

What is essential for adopted children, as for all children, is that one parent remains strong and child-centred throughout their childhood, and acts as their reliable primary carer.

And what can children themselves do? One child in foster care in South Africa, Nkosi Johnson, who died at the age of 12 from AIDS, drew his nation's attention to HIV and AIDS, by becoming a national figure and warning against the dangers associated with the virus right up until the day he died, shaming the South African Government for its lack of action to combat AIDS or spend money on drugs to limit the pain felt by sufferers. Few children and young people in the UK have touched the hearts and minds of the nation, unless they have died tragically, and then the main issues highlighted by their deaths have been professional failings rather than the human situations they found themselves in. Children have been influential in the British care movement. In the 1870s, a boy called Carrots, so-called because of his red hair, knocked on the door of a Barnardos orphanage but was turned away because of a lack of space. The next day, Dr Thomas Barnardo discovered that Carrots had died of exposure out on the street. From that moment, Dr Barnardo vowed never to turn away any child who came to him looking for help.

In her contribution to this chapter, Karen Irving discusses the needs of children with special needs who are often defined as hard to place. Joanna Corbett describes the steps to take in order to successfully recruit adopters. Shelley Mann describes what it was like for her as a child in care forming new attachments within her extended family. Felicity Collier highlights good practice in adoption work today. Phillip McGill asks us not to forget about kinship care. Penelope Welbourne discusses the relevance of attachment theories to the successful parenting or re-parenting of children. Chris Purnell recalls the lifelong impact of his own mother's adoption. And to begin, Kirsty Fergusson tells how she came to be looking after, and loving, as a single parent, a sibling group of four adopted children.

References

Argent, H. (1998), *Whatever happened to Adam?* London, BAAF.

Argent, H. and Kerrane, A. (1997), *Taking extra care – respite, shared and permanent care for children with disabilities*, London, BAAF.

BAAF Adoption and Fostering (2000a), *Surveying adoption, a comprehensive analysis of local authority adoptions in 1998–9*, London, BAAF.

BAAF Adoption and Fostering (2000b), *Linking children with adoptive parents*, London, BAAF.

BBC (2000), *Love is not enough: the journey to adoption*, London, BBC Publications.

Brighton and Hove Area Child Protection Committee (2001), *Part 8 review into circumstances surrounding the death of John Anthony Smith*, Brighton, Brighton and Hove Council.

Broad, B., Hayes, R. and Rushforth C. (2001), *Kinship care for vulnerable young people: identifying good practice and policy*, York, Joseph Rowntree Foundation.

Byrne, S. and Chambers, L. (1997), *Hoping for the best*, London, BAAF.

Byrne, S. and Chambers, L. (1998), *Joining together*. London, BAAF.

Byrne, S. and Chambers, L. (2001), *Waiting for the right home*, London, BAAF.

Cameron, H. (2000) (30 November), *Attachment and trust*, Speaker's paper, Coram Family and Coram Chambers, Inner Temple Hall, London.

Department of Health (2001), *National standards for adoption*, London, Department of Health.

Fitzgerald, J. (1983), *Understanding disruption*, London, BAAF.

Foxon, J. (2001), *Nutmeg gets adopted*, London, BAAF.

Ivaldi, G. (2000a), *Surveying adoption: a comprehensive analysis of local authority adoptions 1998–1999 (England)*, BAAF, London.

Ivaldi, G. (2000b), *Children and families in the voluntary sector: an overview of child placement and adoption work by the voluntary adoption agencies in England 1994–98*, London, BAAF.

Kunstal, F. (1998), *Seven qualities of therapeutic parents* (training material provided for Adoption UK, Banbury, Oxfordshire).

Lidster, C. (1995), *Chester and Daisy move on*, London, BAAF.

Lowe, N., Murch, M. and Copner, R. (2002), *The plan for the child: adoption or long-term fostering?* London: BAAF Adoption and Fostering.

1

ADOPTION'S RICH TAPESTRY UNFOLDED

A family life in the 21st century

Kirsty Fergusson

A desert of sand and stone stretches away to a milky horizon beneath an empty sky of impossible blue vastness. From the right of the picture, a tiny jeep appears, moving slowly, in a cloud of dust, across the landscape. You can just catch a thread of song rising from the jeep: children's voices, shrill and unmelodious, piercing the shimmering heat. Now we're right inside the jeep. A woman driving and three small boys bouncing on the seats, are belting out Oasis, in rough accompaniment to a tinny radio. Suddenly the woman brakes. 'Look boys, pyramids!' she exclaims, pointing. It's me. And it's true: there are pyramids in the distance. I'm jumping over the door of the jeep and running across the sand. The running feels effortless. When I stop and look back in order to check that the boys are behind me, I've come much further than I thought. The jeep is far away and the boys are still clambering over the sides, tiny as insects. I start back towards them, waving, but the dust is blowing up between us and I can only just make out their flailing arms and staggering steps. They are shouting at me to come back and I'm running again, but this time it's too slow and their shouts and frantic gestures are obliterated by the thickening gusts of dust and sand.

I can't forget that dream, although it is nearly eight years old. The boys had been with us for about ten weeks. Ten weeks of undiluted noise and energy; ten weeks of passion, protest, anger and excitement. In ten weeks our lives had crashed together: nights of vomiting, diarrhoea and bedwetting, of padding from bed to bathroom with a sleepy, clinging creature in one's arms and curious, cramped, awakenings with small strangers in the bed; mornings suddenly crammed with arguments over plastic things in cereal packets and telly and washing – socks, pants, sheets, t-shirts – mountains and mountains of it. And the mealtimes – when every potato or slice of cake would release a torrent of memories of foster care, family centre, birth mother. They were eight, six and four; they had eighteen years of memories between them, which had to be delivered into our safekeeping. Sometimes the stories did not tally, for Edward, the eldest, had been fostered separately from his younger siblings. Then violent disputes broke out, which we were unable to pacify with the truth, for neither I, nor my husband, had been a part of their young lives until they came to live with us. Luke, the four-year-old, cried when the tales of violence and neglect were told and begged them to stop. Toby, the middle child, seemed to relish the nasty stuff and encouraged Edward to exaggerate. And they all loved their mother with a desperate fierceness, blaming her circumstances and the company she kept for their own situation. They never blamed her. That unconditional love was astonishingly moving. And it pricked me with anxiety too.

But it was the summer and we lived deep in the country and while the washing flapped on the line they played and fought and ate and ate and made friends with the children of neighbours of whose existence we had scarcely been aware. Social workers came and registered their approval; a year later we all trundled up to the county court and a few minutes later we were their legal, adoptive parents. Because of the history of violence and abuse in the birth family, contact was ruled out. Just one letter a year, with photos to be sent by me to social services, who would forward them on to their mother. There's a photo of us picnicking in the garden with friends. We look like a real family. People who have just met us express genuine surprise when they learn the children are adopted. In a funny sort of way, we've started to look and sound like each other and have adopted the same gestures and mannerisms. I wonder if we've adopted the children or they've adopted us; at any rate, it's clearly a two-way process.

In the photos it looks easy. Friends tell us we're amazing, they couldn't have done it. But photos are deceptive, it's not easy. The photos are like icebergs: you don't see the 90 per cent below the water. Schooling is a nightmare. Living in the country, when everything they want to do takes place in town, eight miles away, is a nightmare. Squabbling, bedwetting and birthday parties leave us exhausted. Toby screams in his sleep for his birth mother, Edward sobs because he has promised his birth mother that when he is eighteen he will return to live with her; Luke clings to the door handle when I'm in the loo. I seem to be doing a lot of smacking and shouting. My husband and I are arguing. He goes to the pub every evening and our dinner sits in the oven, uneaten. Nothing could have prepared us for this. We had made the decision to adopt an older, sibling group after fifteen mostly amiable years together, eleven of them married. Our life of career building and travel followed by a move to the country had been good, but not enough. We wanted a family. Our failure to conceive was unexpected and traumatic and needed swift counter-action. We ruled out IVF and baby adoption on the grounds of too much uncertainty, considered adopting a child from a foreign country briefly, but discarded that idea when we were informed of the costs involved and decided that, as we both liked the idea of sharing our lives with youngsters – rather than babies – adopting a sibling group of older children was the answer. We were interviewed, left to stew, interviewed again and finally the vetting and training procedures got under way. The preparation was inadequate, but then, as I have so often asked myself, what kind of training could ever have prepared us adequately for what was to come? Within a couple of weeks of our approval for adoption, our social worker was presenting us with a case history of the boys. Two months later they were living with us.

At the end of that long and tumultuous summer, my husband was due to go to a conference in Marrakesh. A week before he left, I suggested the boys and I come too. I was afraid of being left on my own with them. In that first year he was calm and kind with them and I was sure he loved them. For this was my private worry: I did not think the adoption could succeed without love and I did not know if I loved them or not. I knew I cared about them and that whatever maternal instincts I had were being exploited to the full; I knew they were all three sparky, special children, immensely likeable and fun as well as hard work. But I didn't know if I loved them. Until I had that dream, the night before we left for Marrakesh and I woke up, weeping and panic-stricken but utterly certain that I loved them.

I look back on photos of that trip with awe and sadness. Blond and brown, in striped shorts bought by their foster parents, they look back at the camera with absolute trust in their eyes. There's a picture of my husband holding Luke close to him, tenderly; Luke's head is bandaged and there are seven stitches above his eye from where he fell against the edge of the swimming pool on the last day. There's me, in the same pool with Toby, laughing, and Edward, in a huge pair of sunglasses that he thinks are very cool, grinning widely. And there's a picture of them caught in a moment of panic, clutching at each other's arms as a snake suddenly rises out of a basket in the market place at Djemma El Fna.

The boys had a younger sister, Didi, who had remained with her mother at the time of their adoption, in the hope that, with help and sound back-up from social services, the relationship would survive. She was a full sister to the youngest boy, Luke. Edward and Toby had a different father. Three years later, to the dismay of the social workers, the little girl, now aged four, was facing the same dangers and neglect as her brothers had experienced and she was placed in foster care. Didi now had two baby half-sisters as the children's mother had formed a relationship with a man who was proving every bit as violent and unstable as the boys' birth fathers had been. I wanted to adopt Didi very much; my husband blew hot and cold about the idea.

For those three years had changed us irrevocably. My husband's business partnership had disintegrated acrimoniously and he was struggling to cope with unemployment and the chaos of life at home. Having more or less abandoned work for the first year of the adoption, I, on the other hand, found myself picking up a career in journalism and running a small but lucrative company from home as well as thoroughly immersing myself in motherhood. I felt confident and strong at a time when my husband felt neither. He began drinking heavily and started seeing another woman. Eventually, he agreed, in a drunken fit of enthusiasm, to adopt Didi, and so she came to live with us, too. The children's birth mother wanted her to live with us, the social workers did not care to look at the iceberg below water level and I did not care to think about the state of our marriage. Didi's adoption went through the court in less than a minute.

Didi, like her brothers, was an extremely beautiful child and had a strong and forthright personality. Just as well, we all said, she'll need to keep her end up with three big, boisterous brothers. But it pole-axed the family. She and Luke were like twins reunited after a three year interval. Physically and temperamentally they were identical. Edward and Toby loathed her and formed a coalition of hatred, never missing an opportunity to attack their sister, both verbally and physically. Mealtimes became minefields; the school run broke down when participating parents were unable to withstand the violence and viciousness of the attacks on the little girl; holidays, when they were incarcerated together in tents, cars, trains or hotels, were intolerable. Before Didi's arrival, the boys had been a tight unit in which Luke's status as half-brother had seemed irrelevant. Now it seemed we were raising two quite different families under one roof, who were at war with each other. Poor Luke, who worshipped his older brothers, felt completely torn down the middle. My husband adored his new daughter and allowed his relationship with the two older boys to turn sour. With Toby in particular, a frightening hostility broke out between them and appalling things were said and done. Our marriage foundered in a terrible atmosphere of regret and contempt. Finally, he left and, after sixteen years of marriage, we were divorced.

And in a funny way, that is where the whole story of this adoption began to make sense for me. All adoptions have their origin in a trauma in which loss and rejection are key ingredients. Amputated from my past life, from a partner who had been 'my other half' since the age of nineteen, I no longer felt like the strong and competent jeep driver in the dream. Although we continued, somehow, to function as a family in which I was more than ever the indispensable provider and anchor, the ultimately incomprehensible loss of a husband and father made us all amputees.

But suddenly, it seemed, the children were more experienced and resilient than me. They, after all, had had to come to terms with the loss of their birth mother, separation from the foster parents who had provided security and stability for three crucial years before they came to live with us, and so, losing their adoptive father fitted an all-too familiar pattern. Didi, in particular, had also lost her two younger half-sisters, who had been adopted by another couple at the same time that she had come to live with us, a couple, who for their own reasons, chose to sever the contact that had been promised and anticipated. And there was my ex-husband, who claimed he had lost me when the children came. There were times when the enormity of our individual and collective losses seemed overwhelmingly disproportionate to what we had gained. Toby began seeing a child psychotherapist because the animosity he was exhibiting towards his sister was intensifying, and this was obviously undermining what seemed like the only good thing to come out of all this loss – that at least the four children 'had each other'. There was only one thing to do, and in the end it happened almost involuntarily, out of sheer self-determining necessity: I let go.

Letting go is the opposite of losing, because in letting go all is to be gained. Letting go is something you choose to do; losing is something that happens to you. I think children, as instinctive creatures, know this better than we adults, who tend to regard their anarchic beginnings with such fear and mistrust. When I say I let go, I mean I let go of the past and I let go of my expectations of the future. The freedom was exhilarating and the children responded with astonishing enthusiasm and acceptance: the old jeep was bumping along again and nobody in it knew where it was going, but we didn't care and we were singing.

We went to live in Spain for four months. Just like that, the winter after my husband and I divorced. It was too wet, too cold, too muddy, too everything and so off we went. The children went to Spanish schools, I took my laptop and carried on writing my weekly columns for the newspapers. We lived by the sea and made new friends. Toby, who had just turned thirteen, hated it; for him it was more losing than letting go. Although initially enthusiastic, he soon resented the loss of his friends, his psychotherapist, his home, even his father. His antipathy for his sister spilled over into terrifying outbursts of anger, which were impossible to control. Didi proved remarkably resilient to these onslaughts, being a tough little character and, like Luke and Edward, maintained that it was 'just how Toby is'. Their sibling love was as unconditional as their love for their birth mother. And for Toby, it proved to be something of a turning point. Forced into the family by our relative isolation in Spain, he had nowhere else to turn, and however appallingly he behaved, and however ghastly the rows and recriminations with me, he was stuck with the fact that we loved him.

One day, I bought an English newspaper, which contained an article supporting the government's new advice to social workers about splitting up sibling groups if it meant adoptive homes could be found more easily for them. I had often wondered if Toby (and the rest of the family) would have been happier if he had been adopted individually and raised as an only child. I had wondered if it we had done the right thing in accepting Didi into the family unit. I read him the article and asked him his opinion. He was careful, but unequivocal in his response. No matter how it appeared, he said, he could not imagine life without his siblings, even Didi. 'All boys hate their little sisters, don't they?' he said. 'But you did the right thing, adopting her, mum.'

The right thing, the wrong thing: I used to live in a world of absolutes in which I knew for certain what was right and what was wrong. It was right for Didi to join her brothers, it was wrong of my husband to desert his family. But so many things which appear to be wrong or right at the time, unleash a chain of events which result in unexpected consequences. I met my husband at London University (good) because I had failed to get into Cambridge (bad); we failed to conceive (bad) but adopted our children (good); the children suffered terrible abuse in their birth family (bad), but would not otherwise have come to live with us (good); our marriage broke down (bad) but I learned the art of letting go (good); and we went to Spain (bad at the time for Toby) but good because it triggered the improvement in his attitude to his sister, from which we have all benefited.

A few weeks ago, to everyone's surprise, we had a phone call from Rebecca, the woman who had adopted the two baby half-sisters. She apologised profusely for the loss of contact and revealed that she had been too afraid to get in touch, as almost immediately after the adoption, her marriage had crumbled and she felt such a failure in contrast to our strong, united and successful adoption and marriage. It was a wonderful reunion: how like each other we had grown, and how easily the children accepted each other. In many ways our experiences and conclusions were parallel, astonishingly so when Rebecca told me that she was taking the little girls to the same island in Spain where we had lived, to further the process of letting go. She had no idea that we had done that, too.

Night. I'm standing in the garden, smoking a cigarette and looking at the old house we have shared for these past eight years. Every window beneath the shaggy thatch is lit and I feel a great surge of affection for this house and its noisy, messy occupants. In his room, Edward is battling with GCSE coursework, trying to find a focus for it in his burning desire to become an army officer. Downstairs, Toby sits at the piano, crooning a love song he has written, playing with two fingers a plaintive melody. Giggles and bubbles escape from an upstairs window: Luke and Didi have invaded the bathroom. On the kitchen table, the remains of a disorderly supper; it appears that the washing-up rota has broken down again. In my office, amid the piles of unfinished articles and photographs, the annual letter I've begun to the children's birth mother. I stick to the facts in these letters and only tell her about the children. 'Edward is now wearing size 13 shoes! He wants to join the army. Toby still very keen on football and tennis. Luke loves making things and fascinated by anything that has an engine. Didi (so tall now) loving school and has smothered her room in S Club 7 posters.' One day, if they want to, the children can fill in the enormous blank spaces in these letters. The phone rings. I hope it's my ex, calling to arrange for them to visit him this weekend. The contact is surprisingly warm now; he is also the subject of their unconditional love.

So much has happened, has needed to happen to bring us to this point in the story, which will never have an end or a conclusion, a moral or a message. I don't intend to start looking for one now.

2

TROUBLED CHILDREN AND
HOW TO PLACE THEM

Karen Irving

A quarter of a century ago, two adoption projects were founded to help children who were not then considered for adoption. These children were those with disabilities, children of mixed ethnic origin, part of a brother and sister group or children who were older. Then as now these children were at the bottom of the pile, passed over in favour of the healthy babies and toddlers, for whom there were many more waiting parents than babies or toddlers waiting for them.

At Parents for Children, the first of the two projects, it was assumed that adoption of disabled and older children would not be trouble-free for the new families. We use a model adapted from the work of an American agency called Spaulding for Children, based in Michigan. When the numbers of babies available for adoption reduced during the 1960s and 1970s, attention shifted to some of the thousands of children drifting in institutions. Could these children be placed in families? Spaulding was founded to see if they could. Kay Donley, Spaulding's charismatic director, brought the idea to the UK. As a result Parents for Children was founded, and soon afterwards a Barnardos project in Glasgow. They began to test out whether the success achieved in America could be replicated here in the United Kingdom. (The route taken by many other European countries was to develop services for adoption of infants from overseas. Inter-country adoption was comparatively rare in the UK until the early 1990s.)

The model of placement used by Parents for Children attempts to ameliorate some of the risk of disruption. Each child who needs a new family is a special 'project'. A family placement specialist is assigned to research the child's history, to organise a publicity campaign featuring the child and to prepare the child for the new family. When a family comes forward, a second family placement worker is assigned to prepare the family for the child. The worker who has prepared the family supports the family and child after placement and after adoption. There is an emphasis on empowering the family and supporting their approach to parenting a child.

The consequences have been extraordinary. Thousands of children who would have drifted in care in the UK were found families. Learning from the Parents for Children and Barnardos example, local authorities were inspired to find families for Down's babies and other young children with disabilities, as well as to explore family placement for the older children in their care.

Although the message that adoption is possible for older children and children with special needs has undoubtedly been a beneficial one, it has created the false belief that almost any child can be adopted successfully without sufficient recognition of the framework within which that work needs to be done. In truth, family placement work is highly complex. It is also expensive. A voluntary adoption agency charges between £12,000 and £30,000 to a local authority to undertake placement of a child with a new family. The actual cost of the work of placing a child who is over five years old will be at least 30 per cent more than the fee charged. The harder the child is to place, the higher the subsidy needed. Voluntary adoption agencies have to raise funds from trusts, donations and legacies to keep afloat. Unfortunately, the fees charged are seen as a drain on the local authority budget.

Adoption is expensive because it takes many hundreds of hours to complete the tasks involved. Careful preparation of both the child and the prospective family and support after placement are essential. The continuity of a link with experienced professionals working within an agency which is open, friendly and knows each family well is vital if families are to care, successfully, for children who have been neglected and abused in early childhood or who have a severe disability.

The fundamentals of good family placement work are proper knowledge of the child, a thorough understanding of the history and functioning of the prospective family, positive endorsement of the family's capacity to be parents, financial support sufficient for the child and family's needs, and an enduring link with experienced social workers, psychologists, therapists and educationalists, among others, so that the child and family can get the support they need when they need it.

Traditionally, Parents for Children has not had a pool of waiting adopters who have been assessed for a theoretical child. Families have come forward in response to a specific child they have seen featured in a publicity campaign. The family has then been prepared for that child, and as they have learned about him or her we have learned about them: their unique history, their strengths and their foibles. It is a method that works well. The family can make sense of our questions about sex because they know that the child has been abused sexually. The assessing social worker facilitates meetings with significant people in the child's life (though rarely with the child at this stage). Some of the pitfalls of the standard assessment process are avoided. We go beyond learning about the family's history in isolation: we learn instead about their response to aspects of the child's history and needs. An important part of the process is accepting them as a unique family and giving them the confidence to care for the child they have chosen. The trust which develops between the family and the social worker is important when it comes to supporting the family after placement.

What constitutes proper and sufficient knowledge of the child? The child's history must include neonatal history, including wherever possible the health records of birth parents. In practice, medical knowledge about the birth father is often unavailable. Medical history is important because, as well as information about the child's medical needs, it contains clues which help us to understand the child's behaviour. Sarah's story illustrates the importance of this. Sarah was placed by her local authority at 14 weeks old with an experienced foster carer. Information about Sarah was scant. She wasn't feeding well. There was thought to be some developmental delay. Sarah's most obvious problem was a persistent, ear-splitting screaming, and one which persisted until Sarah was 2½.

The local authority in charge of placing her had had problems finding a home for Sarah. The daughter of a mother who was of white and Asian origin and an African-Caribbean father, it was thought she should go to a black family. None had been found. When a previous foster placement fell through, Angela (not her real name) agreed to take her at short notice. Nearly six years later, Sarah was referred to Parents for Children with a request to find a permanent family which matched her ethnicity. There was also an implication that Angela was not caring adequately for Sarah. The evidence for this centred round Sarah's somewhat agitated behaviour, isolation from her peers, poor eating habits and low school achievement.

It was not easy to fill in the gaps of Sarah's background and the circumstances of her birth. The Parents for Children worker pieced together information from the local authority's numerous files; hospital records were tracked down. It transpired that Sarah's mother, who we knew had had a history of schizophrenia, was an alcoholic, on drugs and worked as a prostitute. She had stopped taking heroin when she was eight months pregnant. Sarah, however, had been born prematurely.

It became clear that Sarah's early development had been profoundly affected by her mother's addictions, coupled with the chaotic life she had experienced for the few weeks she was with her mother. Far from being the 'normal' baby her local authority social workers had thought her to be, she had probably suffered a considerable degree of subtle but profound neurological damage. Hence the screaming and difficulties in bonding, which led later to uneasy relationships with other children and her carer as well as her struggle to cope in school. Sarah's history is not untypical of the children who need new families. Exceptionally, she had had very few moves during her time in care.

Our understanding of children like Sarah has been helped by the work of neuroscientists who have, in recent years, studied the effects of neglect, chaos and abuse on the developing infant brain. Among the neuropsychiatric diagnoses associated with childhood trauma are severe depression, attention deficit hyperactivity disorder, dissociative disorder, post-traumatic stress disorder, and various developmental disorders.

The brain is made up of many different systems and areas. Not all of these systems and areas develop at the same time. The brain develops in a sequential fashion, starting from the lowest, most regulatory regions of the brain in the brainstem and continuing through to the more complex areas such as the cortex. To develop the motor systems the child must rock, crawl, walk, run and dance. To organise the limbic areas and develop socio-emotional functioning, the child must have consistent, nurturing relationships. To organise cortical areas involved in language and cognition, the infant must be exposed to complex symbolic information. In other words people must talk to the infant. The healthy development of one brain area is dependent on the healthy development of lower brain regions that takes place earlier in the process. Conversely, damage to the lower brain leads to disordered development of each subsequent area. The brain areas that develop first (that is, those that are responsible for sleep, impulsivity, the fear response, regulation of attention and arousal) are less malleable and less responsive to treatment than areas that develop later such as the cortex – the area responsible for thinking (Perry, 1994).

Sadly, timing of experience is crucial. The child who was emotionally neglected for the first three years and then adopted by a loving, nurturing family will still have problems with attachment, intimacy, social interactions, impulse control and other functions dependent on healthy limbic development. In Sarah's case the neglect and abuse she had experienced in the first weeks of her life had profoundly affected the brainstem and midbrain areas. Her screaming had in all likelihood been a response to the terror that as a tiny baby she could not articulate but which primed her brain chemically and in other ways to be constantly alert to danger. Sarah was then 'programmed' to interpret events in her environment as potential threats.

The most fortunate aspect of Sarah's life had been her foster placement with Angela, who had accepted Sarah, nurtured her and expected little back from her. We embarked on a plan to persuade the local authority that Sarah should remain with her carer. Sarah, who has now been adopted by Angela, will never be completely healed. She will always need extra help; but the course of her life will be immeasurably better than it might otherwise have been.

The events in the child's life are hugely important. We go through file records with a fine toothcomb. Obviously we need to know whether the child has been neglected and abused and in what way they have suffered. By this means we can understand the child and how to prepare him or her for the new family. Wherever possible, we meet with each person who has been significant in a child's life. In this way we were able to find a family for Justin, who had learning difficulties, whose birth father had struggled to look after him but was no longer able to do so. Justin's mother had disappeared. It transpired that one of the classroom assistants was very fond of Justin. She had thought that as a young, single, woman she would not be considered as an adopter. Following preparation and assessment, she successfully adopted Justin.

The child's network of family, friends, neighbours and carers must be explored for possible families. It is harder to find adopters than it was 25 years ago. Faced with the difficulty of recruiting families for children young and old, the trend in the US in recent years has been towards placing children with members of the extended family, particularly grandparents, or with members of the child's network of contacts within the community. Only a minority (somewhere between 12 and 25 per cent) of children adopted in the US within the last five years have been adopted by someone not already known to them – so-called 'stranger adoptions'. There has been a drive to support foster carers adopting the children in their care with the payment of adoption allowances which match the fostering allowances, and other benefits including payment for medical care and therapy.

Adoption agencies working with hard-to-place children in the UK welcomed the introduction of allowances following the Adoption Act, 1976. Subsequent regulations made it clear that the allowances were to be calculated according to the child's needs. Regrettably, many local authorities ignored that and opted instead for means-tested allowances based on the adopter's income. In some quarters there is still a view that adopters should not receive additional financial help. They must adopt for love and not for money. The reality is that love is not enough and that adopters do not benefit financially from the process. Hard-to-place children are costly to look after. Most families who are willing to consider adopting an older or disabled child have limited income. Inadequate allowances, inconsistently available, make it even more difficult to recruit new families, or for existing families to adopt more children. It is to be hoped that new legislation improving allowances will make it easier for a wider range of families, including single parents and people on low incomes, to adopt.

A good assessment of the child should include an assessment of IQ. This is not a negative approach: it focuses on the child's potential. Whether or not a child has a statement of special educational need, which includes a report by an educational psychologist, it is helpful to have an up-to-date assessment of the child's abilities to ensure that expectations are not too high or too low. Strengths can be built on, weaknesses identified and extra help provided to overcome difficulties before they become insurmountable.

Support after placement and after adoption is crucial. In theory, appropriate schooling, medical and therapeutic help for the child should be available locally for the family and child. In practice, negotiations about what is required to maintain the child at school usually require hours of social work time supporting the family in lobbying on the child's behalf. There is usually a long waiting list for therapeutic help. For disabled children there is wide variation in provision from area to area. Any agency placing older children needs a resource bank of professionals it can call upon to advise the family or act on their behalf to secure adequate provision of services. A family caring for an angry child with behaviour problems needs someone who can advise on behaviour management, either directly or indirectly, via the support social worker. It is vital for any adoption and fostering agency to have a resource bank which includes consultant clinical and educational psychologists, adult and child psychiatrists, educational advisers and therapists in a variety of fields.

Any adoption agency which seeks to help hard-to-place children has to be able to handle risk. The task of placing an older child, boy or girl, who has been exposed to neglect and abuse is fraught with anxiety and risk and fear of failure for the child, the new family and the adoption agency. It is disheartening for the child and his or her workers when months of researching the child's networks, campaigning publicity that includes national and regional television, national and regional press, mailings to prospective families and events to attract families fails to bring forward a single family for the child.

The hardest-to-place children are boys over the age of five years old. One 10-year-old boy, David, who had waited many months before he was referred to us, was unimpressed with the dozens of sponsored advertisements we secured for him in a major daily tabloid newspaper. 'Surely', he said after a brief spot on television, 'a family will come forward for me now'. It is our experience, however, that the printed media sometimes works better than television. Indeed, we placed David, then aged 11, with a family who, having seen his advertisement in the newspaper, pinned it up in their kitchen while they decided whether to become parents again after their own children had grown up.

We have now decided that we can only work with a small number of older boys at any one time. We know it may take us up to two years to find a family. We know that, however strong the family, their strength will be tested to breaking point by the child's behaviour, and we know that in material terms alone we, as an agency, will lose many thousands of pounds to achieve and to sustain the placement. The child invariably thrives in the new family, unaware that his or her persistent lying, stealing, refusal to wash, inability to concentrate, aggression towards his peers and alarming sexual behaviour present problems to its new parents and can undermine good marriages and life-long friendships.

We often wonder if we have been right to place the child. The strain on good, experienced family placement workers is enormous. The tensions permeate the whole of the organisation, and we dread the possibility that a placement may break down. On the other hand a disruption rate that is very low carries the implication that we are not helping enough of the high-risk children who need help (Barth *et al.*, 1988).

Why do we do it? Simply because agencies like ours see ourselves as the only hope for a small but growing number of children who wait, who long, for a family. But we wonder, daily, if we have made a mistake in our assessment of a child's ability to live in a family. We agonise over whether we have prepared the child and the new family sufficiently well for the task ahead. We worry endlessly whether an episode of abuse by the child will threaten members of the new family, such as grandchildren, or whether the child will allege mistreatment or sexual abuse by his or her new family. We also worry about whether we will be accused of failure if we do not find a match for the child within a reasonable number of months.

As Howe (1998) puts it: 'Adoption practitioners are condemned to choose . . . weighing the strength of one set of facts against another . . . with compassion and humility.' He adds: 'Social practices are irredeemably moral and political practices, which though heavily informed by science, have, in the final analysis, to be conducted using the art of sound argument.'

References

Barth, Richard P. and Berry, M. (1988), *Adoption and disruption*, New York, Aldine de Gruyer, Hawthorne.

Howe, David (1998), Adoption outcome research and practical judgement, *Adoption and Fostering*, 22(2).

Perry, Bruce D. (1994), Neurobiological sequelae of childhood trauma: PTSD in children, in Murburg, M. M. (ed.), *Catecholamine function in post-traumatic stress disorder: emerging concepts*, Washington DC and London, American Psychiatric Press.

3

RECRUITING PARENTS FOR HARD-TO-PLACE CHILDREN

Joanna Corbett

As a social worker working with prospective adoptive parents, I often ask them to describe their 'ideal' child. He, or most commonly, 'she' (as sadly, girls are almost always preferred) will be white, healthy, and have not suffered the lasting effects of emotional, physical or sexual abuse and they are almost always also 'as young as possible'.

Placing children for adoption would be an easy task, if only such children required adoptive families. Back in the 1950s and 1960s, such children outnumbered prospective adopters, and any child outside this category would almost certainly be brought up in residential or foster care. Today, the large majority of children requiring adoptive families do not carry the characteristics of most adopters' ideal child. They tend to be older, have brothers or sisters with whom they hope to be placed, have multiple problems in terms of developmental delay or long term medical uncertainties and suffer the aftermath of abuse of all kinds. Furthermore, we now recognise how important it is to place children, whenever possible, in families who share their culture and ethnicity. Matching these features, again makes the 'ideal' adoptive family harder to find.

Although this sounds a dismal picture, great progress has been made by adoption agencies over the last twenty years in finding excellent adoptive families for such children. So who are these adoptive parents and how do I go about finding them?

There are primarily two routes into adoptive parenthood. Some prospective parents have thought for many years about the idea of adoption, and approach agencies, simply expressing this wish without a specific child in mind. They will undergo a preparation and assessment process over a period of months, working towards approval by that agency as adopters, after which, a link with the 'right' child will be sought. Alternatively, applicants new to the idea of adoption respond to an advertisement for a specific child, perhaps seen as part of an adoption campaign in their local community, or in a newspaper, journal, or television programme.

Whichever way prospective adopters begin their route to adoption, the process of preparation and assessment is essentially the same. It is a thorough, necessarily intrusive, hopefully educational process, which enables prospective adopters to explore their motives to adopt and to examine their potential strengths and weaknesses. This process, known as the home study, entails a series of interviews with a social worker and usually preparatory groups with other prospective adopters where concepts central to adoption are considered. Personal and family referees are also interviewed, statutory checks including full medicals are undertaken, and finally an extensive document known as the Form F is compiled by a social worker, with the prospective applicants. This is presented for consideration by an agency's adoption panel. The panel comprises a range of people including social work professionals, a medical and legal adviser, and others in associated professional fields, but, most importantly, others with a real experience of adoption, either as adoptive parents or adoptees. Many panels now encourage applicants to attend when their application is considered.

Much of my time as an adoption social worker is taken up recruiting a family for a specific child or children who are deemed to be 'hard to place'. So how do I achieve this? My first task is to understand something of the child or children for whom I am seeking a new family. I find it essential to have met the child concerned and to talk to the person who really knows that child – usually their foster carers who know their attributes, habits, problems and general temperament. These impressions, combined with any professional contribution, perhaps from social workers, teachers, or therapists, help to form a pen picture of the child or children I am about to advertise. I also like to form an impression for myself, of how the child makes me feel and also to help the young person, to the best of their ability, contribute in their own way, their thoughts and feelings about their prospective new family.

This is a huge responsibility and it must feel terrifying for any child to think that I am in control of finding their new family. A child has a right to understand what my role is in their life and I have a duty to help this child understand why photographs are being taken, videos made and sometimes why they are appearing on television. Only when a child is very young can this whole process take place without such awareness. Children often provide me with a list of wishes for their futures like 'living by the sea, having two dogs, huge bedrooms, lots of money, toys, trips out', etc, but they often talk of wanting 'someone who will listen to me' and 'somewhere where I won't have to move on'.

So having gathered opinions from all parties involved in a child's life, I write an advertisement, usually limited to a couple of hundred words, which has to describe a child's history, their needs and convey something of what makes them special. A good photograph is absolutely essential. Prospective adopters often say they were attracted to 'something' they saw in a child's face or expression, far more so than to the written word in a short advert.

Publications such as *Be My Parent, Adoption Today* and *Foster Care* magazines, feature such advertisements four or five times per year. These publications go out to those prospective adoptive parents (or current foster carers) who are seeking to adopt. They do an excellent job of linking children with families, but do not attract the many prospective adoptive parents who are not yet linked into the system of adoption. This is why advertising in the wider media becomes so important. For example, a recent opportunity to feature five siblings under the age of 10 on breakfast television attracted an exceptional response of over 150 prospective adoptive families. Advertising the same children in adoption publications brought a minimal response.

Advertising in the media is however, a complex, and difficult process. It is essential to respect children's confidentiality and to be sensitive to their birth family. It is therefore often not possible to provide accurate details about the child's history. Words such as 'neglect' or 'abuse' are often replaced with 'a difficult beginning' or 'experiencing many disruptions'. Social workers learn to decode the language and translate, but I'm not sure many prospective adoptive parents find it that easy.

It is essential that on the day or week that the child is publicised (however that may be), I am available to speak with respondents, if not immediately, always on the same day. I never underestimate the courage people need in making 'that call' to an agency. Positive first impressions are vital. A courteous, interested member of an administrative team who takes accurate messages and assures the caller of my response is essential. When I phone back, I note vital information and ask the caller to explain something of their interest in adoption and why they are interested in this specific child. I then need to convey something of the child's needs, talk more about their history, and let the caller know what will happen next. If they are already linked with an adoption agency and are approved adopters, I ask to speak with their social worker, and perhaps obtain a copy of their Form F. When advertising specific children, I usually place a deadline on responses, quite often a month, after which time I assess the response and decide how to proceed next. An unexpectedly good response is hard to manage.

Quite often a shortlist is drawn up on arbitrary factors such as 'being within a hundred mile radius' or only considering applicants of a certain age range. Inevitably, prospective adoptive parents find such decisions frustrating, especially when they have invested emotionally in the idea of the child or children becoming part of their family. Accompanied by the social worker responsible for the child, we then usually visit prospective families and during the course of probably just one interview, have to decide if this family could meet the needs of my specific child. Similarly, the family must decide if they would like to become this child's adoptive parents. Sometimes I find myself in the difficult but fortunate position of being able to choose between a number of prospective applicants. Alternatively and more usually, for hard to place children, my task is to assess if the positives of perhaps only one potential family outweigh risk factors which may also be evident. Sometimes other compromises have to be reached. Many prospective adopters of former years choose now to foster instead, attracted by the payment of a reasonable allowance for a difficult task, and knowing they will always 'share' responsibility for the child with others. Sometimes I have to accept that applicants offering the permanent legal security of adoption cannot be found for some children, and accept that a good foster family is the 'next best' option.

So what kind of applicants successfully adopt hard to place children? The most essential criteria is that applicants can really accept the child or children as they are now, not as they hope they may become. This becomes particularly relevant when a child is half way through childhood, or has disabilities or emotional difficulties which may be slow or very difficult to resolve. Such children test out even the strongest of relationships so it is essential that applicants in partnerships are equally united in their motivation to adopt and that their relationship is strong. Single adopters often cope really well with hard to place children and although their practical pressures may be greater, they often comment that they do not have anyone other than the child or children to consider. I also seek applicants who are easy going, but have some sense of routine to their lives, a sense of humour and good support networks, and who are not anxious about being different from others.

There are some common misconceptions about adoption, such as you have to be under 40 years old, you can't adopt if you already have children, or that you won't be considered if you are divorced or have been in care as a child yourself. Often the most appropriate adopters of hard to place children are experienced parents whose children are now in their late teens or twenties. Similarly, when adopters' life experiences have brought separation and loss, they often have a greater potential to understand and help cope with the pain in a child's life.

Assuming a prospective match between adoptive family and child has been made and the link formally approved by the child's adoption agency, the sensitive process of introduction begins. Usually, over a period of weeks, depending upon the child's age and individual needs, the prospective adoptive family and their chosen child meet and begin to develop a relationship. The first visit usually takes place in the child's current placement – home territory where the child feels more in control. It is an exciting, difficult occasion. Both parties are nervous and have high expectations and inevitably both are frightened that the link won't be right. I have learnt over the years that first impressions should not be ignored, and almost always mirror the eventual outcome of a future placement. Sadly, some applicants know immediately that the link isn't right whilst others feel convinced from the first moment they saw their child that they were meant to be a family. For others there is some ambivalence, but a glimmer of possibility in that first meeting.

Older children almost always know their own feelings about their prospective new parents, and will make these clear, either verbally or non-verbally. For prospective adoptive parents this can be harder. They often wonder if love will grow or they begin to feel guilty about ambivalence, or jealous of their partner who appears to feel more enthusiastic than they do. My role is help make sense of these emotions while the child's social worker decides if the match seems right from the child's perspective.

If the first meeting has gone well, the introductory process continues, aimed at the development of relationships. The child and family spend increasingly longer together and eventually the child will spend time, including overnight stays, in their new home before finally moving to their new family. Next, the long process of adjustment and learning to live together begins. The honeymoon period is a common feature in adoptive placements – new adopters often wonder why the former carer found the child so 'difficult' or why social workers were so 'negative'. They congratulate themselves on how well they are coping and how much easier everything feels than they had envisaged. When this pattern is evident, I always remind adopters that when, and if, things change they will have these happier memories to lean on, knowing that there is hope for the future!

Almost always, once a child has really settled, and dares to trust and convey something of the anguish of their often unsettled lives, their behaviour will become more difficult and adopters will need help to hold on and find new strategies of coping. In the early weeks of a placement I usually visit a family weekly or fortnightly, decreasing when appropriate. However, when problems occur, adoptive families need close and immediate support of the social worker who knows them well, not just an out of hours emergency number for social services.

As months pass and hopefully the child begins to feel settled, the time has come for the prospective adopters to lodge their adoption application with the court. This can be a stressful period, especially when the adoption application is to be contested by a child's birth parents and may be protracted. However, the granting of an adoption order always brings a sense of finality to the whole family. Adopters often express immense relief at this stage and some say they didn't realise how they were holding back some of their feelings until their adopted child becomes 'really theirs'.

Although this marks the formal ending to my involvement with families, post-placement support is an essential part of the adoption process. Often years later, families may reach a crisis in their family lives, and will need professional guidance, or reassurance. Many agencies offer regular informal events such as adopters' picnics, training sessions and so on, which facilitate a continuity of contact and enable them to make relationships with other families like their own.

In conclusion, the placement of hard to place children is a fascinating, complicated and risky process. Much can go wrong along the way, but to see a child blossom, both physically and emotionally, and to see the satisfaction adoptive parents feel brings job satisfaction beyond any measure.

4

IT CAN ONLY GET BETTER,
AND IT DID!

Shelley Mann

Passed from pillar to post for my first two years of life, in foster care from the age of two to twelve years, orphaned and then two years later adopted at the age of fourteen – this all seems a little harrowing when first heard. However, having only known stable foster care, and being fortunate enough that my newly acquired family were, in fact, all related to me as my paternal aunt and uncle and cousins, who became my sisters, eased the blow – at least for me anyway.

I was born Michelle Evans and in August 1974, when I was nearly two, I was made the subject of a care order to Cheshire County Council. To ensure that I would still be cared for by my family, my paternal aunt and uncle, Meg and Geoff Mann, applied to become my foster parents. My natural parents, Sue and Paul Evans, were extremely vulnerable, due to heavy drug abuse and so were unable to manage their lives and relationships with consistency, which led, at two years old in December 1974, to my foster placement within the Mann family.

Regular contact with Sue and Paul was anticipated and actively encouraged from the outset, taking into account the difficulties they both had in maintaining consistent attitudes and keeping to agreed plans. But it wasn't uncommon for them to be so out of it that they would generally forget arranged meetings, or fail to understand that a care order was, in reality, the safest and best option for me.

They eventually lived separate lives: Sue drifted into different relationships, and Paul fought his drug dependency with limited success. With the support of his sister, Meg, he was able to spend more time with me than Sue could and for a time lived near us in Hertfordshire at a local hostel. I was able therefore to establish a close relationship with him until I was almost seven years old. But in October 1979 he died following a drug overdose. The inquest reached an open verdict, and I was left with the fond memories of my childhood that I was fortunate enough to share with him.

45

I was very upset about Paul's death and for a while was unable to settle, experiencing nightmares but generally took it in my stride, as I had imagined all seven-year-olds would tend to do. I encountered for the first time the different approaches that people would take towards me as a child labelled as growing up in care and experiencing a parent's death at such an early age.

I was able to distinguish between these approaches and used them to my advantage. For example, I was extremely aware that I could be naughty at school and would not be in trouble, as allowances would be made 'due to her circumstances'. That was all very well, but circumstances do change, sometimes for better or worse, but the attitudes stayed the same. The softly-softly approach was all very well, fantastic for manipulation, but it can all too easily used as an excuse for children who veer off the rails.

More credit should be given for the intelligence of children, as it is all too easy to patronise and tread lightly, when plain honesty would suffice and keep them on track. No child wants to go down the self-destruct road. I certainly didn't and was entirely aware of the tight safety nets and boundaries that had been set, as I tried to break them, each in itself a test for my foster family and my relatives.

Sue's reaction to Paul's death was immediately to regain an interest in my welfare, although still unable to maintain any consistency in her contact with me. She began to talk of regular visits to establish a closer relationship again but unfortunately her enthusiasm was short lived and after arranging to visit me on my birthday, less than a month after Paul's death, she failed to turn up, without an explanation, as she had on previous occasions.

Sue's unreliability was a cause for concern as I was far more aware of my relationships and identity within the foster family and was becoming sensitive to the fact of having two mums. Everything was pretty volatile: I was seven years old, extremely angry and confused and knew even then that she was running away and avoiding the situation. I was also aware that Meg and Geoff were finding it hard to conceal their hostility towards her. Enough became enough. Even at seven years of age you didn't have to be Sherlock Holmes to work that one out. Yet despite these complications in my life I still had the ability to make the most of any given situation and maintain my personality.

My anger and frustration over the next few years was fuelled by my bewilderment at Sue's ability to flit in and out of my life unceremoniously. I began to recognise the differences between my two mums and, in retrospect, I can see that Sue was living a complete fantasy – one I could only participate in when she would eventually visit me, thus knocking down and destroying the tight safety nets and boundaries that had been carefully laid down by Meg. As I tried to break them, each action in itself was a test for my foster mother, who stood for everything stable and secure in my life, whether I liked it or not, and I certainly did not.

By now I was beginning to feel an overwhelming disapproval towards Sue and her way of life, and how her actions were affecting mine. I had a newfound awareness, opened up by seeing the harsh reality of Sue's way of life. For example, the different partners she had were men more unreliable than she was. I am very grateful for a visit to see her in Manchester, to see her and her new partner in their new flat. It turned out to be another eye-opener. I couldn't rip away the pedestal from underneath her quickly enough; her true colours were not unexpected, but I had at least hoped my worst fears would have been wrong.

Sadly there was no denying the truth, that there was no way my natural mum was at all capable of looking after herself, let alone me. In hindsight, contact with Sue was a springboard into uncertainty and insecurity each time. I had a well-established position within my foster family, and was quite aware of the reasons why I was there. Meg and Geoff had always been openly regarded as mum and dad, and my natural parents were known as Mummy Sue and Daddy Paul. This suited everyone and helped ease any doubt about having two sets of parents. It especially helped me to feel part of the family, as my foster sisters called them mum and dad so why would I want to differ? It seemed a natural process and assumption, and especially stopped confusion at school. When I started secondary school I used the Mann surname to avoid any more confusion as I was known as the youngest sister of the Mann family and naturally acted and was treated as that.

The negative feelings I had harboured towards Sue were ready to come out at last. About time, I thought, having spent the last ten years gradually filtering them through into words. And so, in July 1984, at an arranged visit to see her in London, where she was then living, I told her how it was. I was no longer a two-year-old and wanted her to stop thinking of me as such. I had grown up and expected honesty and a reasonable commitment to the contact I had with her. I also challenged her drug addiction. I felt extremely relieved that I was able to have a frank discussion with her and that she had at least listened and understood my comments.

At last I felt that our relationship now had a basis of reality and truth on my terms rather than the fantasy she had created and wanted me to participate in. I felt we were entering a new era. Having taken a deep breath and blown away the cobwebs, I could now look forward to building a new relationship with my mother, and possibly her new partner, Joe, who, she assured me, was not the same as the others. I had my doubts which were to be tragically confirmed. Six months later, in December 1984, whilst living in East London, Sue was murdered by Joe. He was found guilty of manslaughter and sentenced to eight years imprisonment.

This shook the whole family, and opened up a whole new can of worms. The first feeling was relief and the guilt that came with it. I was extremely aware of the relief and guilt that I felt when the news was broken to me. I felt the atmosphere of the family's apprehension as to what my reaction was going to be. I wasn't sure of my reaction and so placed it on hold, and found it hard to watch my foster family's reactions. The responsibility I had carried felt like it had been confirmed. I sought comfort within my cousins or sisters as I had come to regard them, and ironically, they mothered me to a certain extent, especially Rachel, who chose to put my feelings before her own; when the police arrived, to inform us of Sue's death, she became very distressed on my behalf.

In response to her caring and motherly nature, I retaliated by challenging her emotions, and accused her of being a fraud. With the power of hindsight I can see that she was trying to protect me, yet I had interpreted the reality that she was closer to her uncle Paul than she was to her aunt Sue as a direct challenge to my own emotions. I felt a strong sense of sibling rivalry until I realised that if this was my way of dealing with things, it wasn't doing anyone, let alone me, the least bit of good. I realised that sibling support was a much better option, and welcomed all that was going.

For Meg, Paul's death had been particularly painful; she knew she was vulnerable following Sue's death and was frank in sharing with the family the demands that her own grief along with mine would make upon us all. This in itself was a definite strong point for the family, as we could all be as frank as possible, knowing that honesty was the best policy, and this without a doubt, was the case within the family. Dishonesty was not tolerated, and I knew therefore the buttons to press when I wanted to gain attention, or show signs of insecurity. This consisted of petty theft around the home, followed by denial, and it was a favourite of mine whenever I needed to test the care and security of the family unit.

Sue's death was significant in my regaining contact with her own family. Following my placement with Meg and Geoff, I had had no contact with my maternal grandparents and many aunts and uncles. I met the family at my mother's funeral, and was warmly received. Obviously I was overwhelmed at the discovery of such a large number of relatives, and was tempted by the thought of frequent visiting.

Aunt Marilyn was particularly significant in offering information about Sue. We wrote from time to time and I spent a weekend with her in 1985. Communication with the family in Manchester, however, became minimal, and it was mutually agreed as appropriate since they had been assured that I was fine and doing well. After meeting such a vast and friendly family in the north, I became aware of new options that had not been issues until my discovery of this new and exciting side to my life.

I was now an orphan. I was 12 years old. What was to become of me now? What if this new and exciting family wanted to make up for all those years of inattention? Would I still stay with my paternal relatives? These were real issues that made me stop and look at my life and where it had been and where it was going. I had grown up in this family and my emotional and physical development had flourished. My position as the youngest child helped me to bond with them and I saw myself as very much one of the family. I was very happy where I was and didn't want to change anything, yet felt that it was somehow not complete. However, if they adopted me, this would secure my place within the family on a permanent basis and on a legal basis.

Great minds thought alike, and I was thrilled to hear that Meg and Geoff held the same views. The adoption application was made. Marilyn and family were also in agreement with the proposed adoption and it all sounded so simple and straightforward, yet none of us had accounted for the hoops of fire that social services expected us to jump through. I saw the adoption application as not changing anything, but just making me legally a member of the Mann family, rather than being an Evans out on my own. I had spent ten years in permanent foster care with this family and considered them to be my family. After all they were my aunt, uncle and cousins.

The whole process took just over two years for the adoption to be finalised. I am still baffled at the length and time and the procedures that were involved, and can remember the frustration experienced as a family over the interviews, forms, discussions, and reports, which were compulsory. We suffered frustration and pressures in what was a major upheaval for us. We had just dealt with the death of my mother, and I was desperate for a sense of belonging and stature. And given my age, my little hormones were bouncing about all over the place, which again didn't help. For me, the drawn out lengthy process of adoption seemed more traumatic than the death of my natural parents – as at least that had a finality about it.

At last, a panel and a judge decided it was a good idea after all that I should be adopted, by the family that I had lived with for twelve years. So on 16th December 1986, almost exactly twelve years after I began to live with them, the application was approved and I was at last legally a member of the Mann family, from then on to be known as Shelley Michelle Mann. If there was one thing that I would never forget about that day, it would be the 'oh-so-out-of-touch-patronising-judge', who exclaimed as we were leaving, 'You must be so happy, you've finally got what you've always wanted?'. 'Not likely matey', I thought, if I had what I had always wanted, it would have been my real parents, and a wonderful family home together. Still, I think I know what he meant to say.

I was very fortunate to have had a nice and understanding social worker who I still remember. She was supportive, and I felt that Hertfordshire Social Services did themselves proud through the care and attention that they gave to me. It is possible to grow up in care and not be damaged by the circumstances that surround you, but for that to happen it takes strength and willpower. I was fortunate to have been fostered and adopted by relatives and experienced the best kind of kinship care available to me at that time.

It wasn't until 1997 that Marilyn, Sue's sister, contacted me again. It was a welcome surprise out of the blue and we now exchange letters and phone calls on a regular basis.

Looking back to my reactions when Sue and Paul died, and the long term effects and implications it caused, I think Paul's death didn't have such an overwhelming effect as might have been expected. I was nearly seven and my understanding of death was quite innocent in my little protected world of the 'seven-year-old', and I knew that this was a 'big one', due to the sadness that I felt and saw within the family. Meg explained it to me as well as she could, and I was aware of the difficulty she had in finding the right words, and admired her bravery as she told me the news of the death of her brother – my father.

Ironically, I compared the situation to the death of our pet rabbit, which I had loved dearly as any child does with their first pet. It had been my friend and a learning curve for the feelings that I was unknowingly going to experience: joy when playing, pain and hate when bitten, and rejection when I couldn't pick him up. Holding the rabbit still in my hands, cold, and definitely not up for a lettuce leaf or two, I made a mental note of the feelings as I knew something special had gone forever, and that it was an important lesson to be learnt. I recalled this lesson when the news of my father's death was broken to me, and felt comforted by it.

Personally, for me, looking back, experiencing death at such a young age of seven years was a case of 'ignorance was bliss'. There were fewer questions to ask at that age. Whilst I look back with sadness, I also feel my knight in shining armour did arrive, in the form of the Mann family. My ability to accept Paul's death, as just one of those things that life was to throw at me, stays with me even now, as I have no regrets or unfinished business with him.

Sue's death affected me far more powerfully than I could have ever had admitted or realised, and woe anyone fool enough or brave enough to try and point it out to me at the time. When I finally took my reaction off hold, and opened the can of worms I had been nurturing for so long, the unfinished business with Sue had transformed itself into some pretty ugly snakes. I chose to ignore the harsh reality that Sue resembled, and cushioned myself in a world of mother like daughter, and believed my own fantasy that things could have and would have worked out in the end.

Meg and Rachel were always my wake up call, and I hated every minute of it, and let them know with my full vengeance. For many years I couldn't even discuss Sue with Rachel, however close I was to her. I was convinced that Rachel hated Sue, resented me, and dismissed her concerns for me as my own sibling rivalry. I was feeling punishment and guilt for stealing her position as the youngest child when I first arrived. This attitude coupled with my regular testing of the tight boundaries, attempted to push everyone to their limits, and thankfully, no matter what I threw at them, the safety net was always in place. I felt extremely alienated at times and couldn't see the wood for the trees, even after the adoption had gone through, and in all honesty, that was when I really demanded full attention, letting my anxiety and self destruct button take over.

I now couldn't feel more secure and part of the Mann family if I tried. All children test their parents, but I felt like I had to be extra sure. Each time I wobbled off the rails, they were there to put me back on, encouraged me through art college, kept a tight reign, and gave me honest support at all times.

I now have the confidence to keep myself on a tight track, and look forward to the testing times that I will experience with my own son Oliver. My own childhood has set firm foundations for my role as a mother, and I am very affectionate, confident and loving towards my son and my partner Darren. I get the balance right, and although I do have very high expectations and values of myself, I am firm and fair. I know these expectations are impossible to achieve, but need them in a sense to remind me of how different I am from my natural mother, and also how like her I am as well.

When I understood her incompetence as a mother, I vowed to never make the same mistakes as her, and to never forsake my children and responsibilities. This resulted in a decision that I would never have a child until I knew in myself that it was the right time. Right, meaning that I had to be in a long-term relationship, and to be secure financially and emotionally. I felt that until I had these foundations in place, I could only then bring up a child properly. Without such a thing life would be very hard indeed, and I certainly wouldn't have been able to negotiate my return to work on a part-time basis, and have Oliver attend day nursery part time.

My sister Clare has been and still is a wonderful sounding board for when my expectations verge upon the scale of neurosis. She has three girls of her own, aged four, six and eight, and in my eyes, has been there, done it and bought the T-shirt with baby sick all over it! This again is another plus at having acquired three sisters, as I am never short of someone to talk things through with.

This support from my sisters came in very handy, over the years, as I refused to grow up and progress, wanting to stay as a child, and was extremely immature for my age. Over the years however, I became aware of the hindrance my childhood had had on me and wanted to mature, and leave my insecurities behind. So I decided that counselling was a sure way forward. Mum and Dad encouraged me to do so and helped me find my 'lady', who was going to listen to me babble on for the next four years. I felt a strong need to piece together the surreal jigsaw that resembled my life and I am certain that counselling helped me become what I am today.

Rachel has always described me as calm waters running deep, and this is very true, as the depth of my childhood will always bring out the white water rapids that I hold within myself, but at least now I am experienced enough to ride them with confidence. I was one of the lucky ones, and now enjoy a happy family life of my own, with my partner Darren, and my lovely son, Oliver.

I do not believe that I could have survived it all alone, and feel that the unconditional love that I experienced within the family helped me through my traumatic childhood. They gave me the strength to confront the ghosts of my past, and be the rounded level-headed person that I feel I have become today.

5

GOOD PRACTICE IN ADOPTION

Felicity Collier

Assessing the suitability of adults to adopt a child is, arguably, one of the most awesome tasks which a social worker faces. The responsibility is enormous – on the one hand, you have a child who is very likely to have suffered abuse and neglect, sometimes of the most appalling nature; this child will also have experienced at least one profound loss in being separated from its birth mother and probably many more, both before and after coming into the care of the local authority. Such children only have social workers to protect their future. They will find it difficult to trust a new family, they may well test them to their limits and for a significant number (probably one in five) the adoption will not work out and the child will be returned, even more lonely and traumatised, back into 'care.'

On the other hand there are the adoptive applicants – often adults who have already experienced the sadness of being unable to have children of their own including the repeated indignities of unsuccessful fertility treatment; now they are putting their heads above the parapet to ask to adopt a child. These applicants will have read in the media the awful stories of intrusive social workers and are steeled to be interrogated about their most personal experiences and terrified of being rejected – rejection could be the final nail in the coffin of their self-esteem if they have failed to conceive and also failed to be deemed suitable to care for a child.

Potential for conflict for social workers in such a situation can only be imagined. They will feel they are the guardians of the child's welfare and will have to try to make the best possible choice for the child in the circumstances. At the same time, they will experience the strength of feeling, the hopes and aspirations of the prospective adopters whose lifestyle and family are likely to be very different to those the child has experienced. It is fortunate that in most social services departments, the task of approving a family and the task of assessing the suitability of an approved family for a particular child's needs fall to different social workers. This too can be part of the problem as it means that inevitably prospective adopters feel they have to jump through two sets of hoops before becoming adoptive parents – the first being the approval process as to their suitability as adopters and the second being their suitability to parent a particular child.

Given the complexity of all of this, it is reassuring to know that the great majority of adopters whose details are placed before an adoption panel do pass this particular hurdle. Indeed, Ivaldi (1999) demonstrated that 94 per cent of these families were approved as adopters. The unknown element, and there is no consistent monitoring of this at present, is the number of prospective adopters who drop out earlier in the process. Given the shortage of families for the sort of children now needing adoption, this information, including the reasons for withdrawal, would be extremely useful.

For the benefit of the reader it is necessary to recap briefly on the process from initial enquiry to adoption. Most potential adopters will approach a local authority or voluntary adoption agency as a result of national or local publicity, or will have contacted the agency to make a preliminary enquiry. They will then receive some written information and should be offered an appointment to discuss their interest further. If they are still interested, and there is no obvious reason why they should be excluded at the outset (for reasons such as lack of availability of the particular children, perhaps infants, that they might wish to adopt), then they will probably be invited next to an information session with other people who have adopted children and subsequently to some preparation group meetings where they will be able to learn more about what adoption might mean for them and their families. If they then decide to make a formal application, references including medical and police checks, will be taken up. They will have a number of meetings with a social worker who will work with them to draw up a report about their circumstances and background, their knowledge and understanding of parenting the sort of children needing adoption and what their particular family and circumstances might have to offer.

Adopters are told: 'The process aims to offer you a full, honest and open assessment. It should provide both you and the agency the opportunity for showing the strength you bring as well as any concerns, and you should be helped to work in partnership with the social worker responsible for your assessment – the aim is to achieve a successful placement for yourself and the child, not simply to be approved (British Agencies for Adoption and Fostering, 1998).

Reports will then be submitted to the adoption panel which will make a recommendation to the nominated decision maker in the adoption agency as to whether approval should be given . If the applicants are unhappy at the recommendation they will be able to make representations to the decision maker in writing and will have access to the complaints procedure.

It all sounds relatively simple but clearly the process is fraught with difficulties along the way – the potential for misunderstanding between social workers and applicants, who may have very different expectations and experiences, is significant. However well-trained and competent the social workers are, it is vital that they are able to recognise the influence of their own personal experiences of family life and to ensure that the view they are able to take is as objective as possible and based only on clear and observable evidence. The recent introduction of a competency model of assessment, where, as well as looking at adopters' social history, there is a focus on the parenting skills they can demonstrate, is potentially a more transparent process. From the adopters' perspective, this may be the first time in their lives that they have met with a social worker and inevitably their own prejudices and anxieties about this can influence the process. They may feel vulnerable and exposed as they talk about very personal experiences in their lives with not only a complete stranger, but someone who may seem to them young and inexperienced and often of quite a different background.

Given all of this, it is refreshing that so many adopters speak so positively of their social worker and find the whole assessment a helpful process – indeed the Prime Minister's own review of adoption found no evidence of blanket exclusions of applicants with particular characteristics. Despite this, there is popular mythology that many loving and suitable adopters are excluded because of age, weight, smoking and so on, or because they are the 'wrong race' or read too many books. It is true that in a small number of cases these factors may be relevant. For example, most people would not think it appropriate for an infant relinquished by its birth mother to be adopted by a couple in their sixties – to have your parents outlive your childhood and to have reasonable energy and good health are not unreasonable expectations for a child who has already lost one family. Equally, to place an infant with parents who smoke, when there is such a wide choice of people available and the health risks of passive smoking are well known, would hardly be the act of a responsible corporate parent.

It has struck me on occasions that if public understanding of the importance of approving adopters could be enhanced there would be more potential adopters and a great deal more confidence and less blame attached to the social work profession. The series of television programmes (*Love is not enough*, BBC1) followed several families through the approval process and viewers said they realised for the first time that these were very difficult decisions. If more families are to come forward and if the community at large is to have respect for social workers on the front line doing this difficult and demanding job, it has to be acknowledged that approving adopters is not a scientific process – indeed Triseliotis noted that 'assessment is an imprecise process because there are no firm criteria of what qualities exactly are required to parent other people's children. Even when we know what to look for it is not always easy to recognise the presence or absence of such qualities as maturity, stability of couple relationships, warmth and capacity for close relationships. Motivation, too, is a difficult attribute to evaluate' (Triseliotis *et al.*, 1997).

Despite the fallibilities of assessment, we cannot replace it by using short cuts or semi-automatic approval. Indeed, following the trial by the media in 2001 of the Kilshaws, who sought to bring into this country for the purposes of adoption infant twins from the US located through the internet, there are few people who do not believe that there is a role for social workers in checking carefully the credentials of all adopters. The challenge for us all now is to build on this greater potential for understanding and to explain to the public what the crucial elements of excellent adoption practice are.

The national standards for adoption services were drawn up by an expert group, which included the Department of Health and people whose personal lives have been directly affected by adoption. The quality of service to prospective adopters has been of critical importance within these standards. The principle is fundamental to the way forward: 'People who are interested in becoming adoptive parents will be welcomed without prejudice, responded to promptly and given clear information about recruitment, assessment and approval. They will be treated fairly, openly and with respect throughout the adoption process.' (Department of Health, 2001).

The standards go on to require that written eligibility criteria are provided for adoptive parents, with full and fair explanation of the assessment and approval process, together with clear, written timescales. Indeed, if the latter alone were addressed there would be tremendous progress. It is simply not good enough that some adopters have to wait up to two years from the beginning to the end of the approval process, a delay often aggravated by a shortage of social workers and delays in completing the necessary checks. Of course, some situations will be more complex and more work will be needed but the intention is that there should be a decision within six months of all formal applications to adopt.

The other major improvement which will make a difference will be the setting up, as included in the Adoption and Children Act, of a transparent appeals process will be run by an independent agency. Many will criticise how resource intensive this will be at a time of tremendous pressure on social workers, but if we remember the heavy investment made by adopters in the whole process and the impact on them personally of putting their lives on the line, then we surely cannot deny them access to an appeal mechanism.

Much emphasis has been put on the importance of establishing an effective partnership between adopters and their agency. However, Murch and Lowe commented:

> assessment ... implies a degree of doubt about suitability, an element that is hard to combine with the notion of partnership. We do not think that you can have successful partnerships when one party is effectively on trial by the other ... As there is a statutory requirement with agencies who supervise a placed child, we do not see how the dilemma can be avoided.
>
> (Murch and Lowe, 1999)

I would suggest that while the notion of partnership can be an empowering one, what is vitally important is for the worker to demonstrate fairness and openness and respect for applicants. Of course there is a power imbalance, but this power imbalance is reflected nowhere more strongly than in the lack of power of the children whose future is at stake.

As we all strive to reduce delays for children, and as targets set by government emphasise the need for quick decisions, perhaps it is fitting to listen to the words of a boy, aged thirteen, who responded to the recent adoption standards consultation. He said: 'but if the right family cannot be found then the children should stay in foster care. The child should be able to choose the family it will be living with for the rest of its life. It should not be made to live with someone it doesn't want to.'

References

British Agencies for Adoption and Fostering (BAAF) (1998), *Understanding the assessment process*, London,

Department of Health (2001), *National adoption standards for England*, London: Department of Health.

Ivaldi, G. (1999), *Children and families in the voluntary sector*, London British Agencies for Adoption and Fostering.

Murch, M. and Lowe, N. (1999), *Supporting adoption: reframing the approach*, London, British Agencies for Adoption and Fostering.

Triseliotis, J., Shireman, J. and Hundleby, M. (1997), *Adoption: theory, policy and practice*, London, Cassell.

6

KINSHIP CARE
A child in the family

Phillip McGill

There are many children who are not looked after children but who are cared for by relatives or friends of their parents (kinship carers), and some children who do become looked after have relatives or friends who put themselves forward to care for them. Most local authority adoption, fostering and permanent placement teams will be supporting some carers who are relatives or friends of the child for whom they are caring. Some of the support work with relative and friend carers will be provided by social workers in child protection and children in need teams.

However, anyone approaching a social services department and asking to be put in touch specifically with the kinship carers, family and friends carers, or residence order carers' teams is likely to be disappointed. Kinship, foster or residence order carers are likely to receive a qualitively different and lower level of support (financial, practical and emotional) from social services.

The invisibility of kinship carers is just one more aspect of the complexity of adoption and fostering. As has been argued elsewhere in this book, the arguments about adoption are not nearly as straightforward as statements by the media and politicians sometimes suggest. Alas, for them rhetoric falls down in the face of the facts. Not the least of these uncomfortable facts is about which children people want to adopt and who comes forward to adopt them. For example, in England there are few people applying to adopt children over five years of age. Most of the people applying to adopt children under the age of five are white and are either stranger carers or step-parents. Few black and ethnic minority people apply to adopt children under five years of age compared with the number of children for whom this is the plan (and where this is not a step-parent adoption).

Some of the children under five and many of the children over that age, may initially have a plan for adoption, but if adopters cannot be found the plan will be reviewed and is likely to be changed to long-term fostering. As well as the significant lack of black adoptive parents and the age of the child, other reasons why adopters cannot be found may be to do with the child's having particular medical or other special needs, or where the child is part of a sibling group to be placed together.

Residence orders are made on the basis of a pre-existing significant relationship between the applicant carer(s) and the child. Most residence order carers are kinship carers.

Those looked-after children who are not rehabilitated with their parents and for whom adopters or residence order carers cannot be found, or where their plan recommends they are not adopted or made subject of a residence order, rely upon the availability of kinship or stranger foster carers who are prepared to look after them in the longer term.

The majority of long-term foster placements are made with stranger carers. These placements have a high disruption rate (where the placement irretrievably breaks down and the child has to move) and consequently many of the children in these placements will experience one or more changes in their placement before they reach the age of sixteen. The disrupting of a placement can have a significantly negative effect upon the child's ability to settle into their next placement.

There is a particular lack of foster placements for teenage children which, coupled with the difficulties these young people have in settling into new foster families, leads to many adolescent children who have had previous disrupted fostering placements being placed within residential care rather than in new foster families. Sometimes residential care is the first choice for a young person because of the their circumstances.

Many residential units, as well as boarding schools, require young people to have a home base with parents, kinship or stranger carers, for the unit's or school's holidays and there is the same lack of availability of these placements. Some looked-after teenagers will run away from their foster or residential placement and will return to their parent's home or to other kinship carers.

Despite these placement shortfalls and shortcomings, we persistently under value kinship and residence order care. This is not merely a question of attitude. In practical terms, the differences in the treatment of stranger foster carers and kinship carers are considerable: where the former kind of carer for an adolescent may receive up to £250 per week as an allowance and have the support of two named social workers (one for the child and one for the carers), the kinship foster carers or residence order carers of the same young person might receive a weekly allowance of up to £80 and have one named social worker (for the child), or no specific support service.

In some other countries, and more recently in England, family group conference projects have become involved in contacting the extended families and friendship networks of some looked-after children and have 'discovered' relatives or friends willing to become involved in caring for the child on some basis. Some of these relatives and friends were unknown to social services and had not been involved in the child's plans before; some had some previous involvement and had chosen not to become involved with social services or had been discouraged by the low level of support offered to them.

Some of the children who have had family group conferences arranged were then placed with the kinship carers identified in the family group conference plan. It is possible that there are other 'looked after' children, currently living with stranger carers, who through the intervention of a family group conference could move to live with kinship carers.

It is important to note that the number and range of stranger and kinship adoptive, foster or residence order placements has never compared well with the number of children, or range of needs of those children, for whom adoption, foster or residence order care is the plan. Social services departments should be doing as much as they can to encourage increasing the number and range of the placements available to looked-after children.

One of the many considerations in relation to promoting kinship care is the respective 'quality' of kinship versus stranger foster care. In some ways, this might be seen as an academic exercise because there are not presently sufficient kinship or stranger carers available.

Sometimes it may be that for one young person there was a choice of an 'inexperienced' kinship carer and an 'experienced' stranger foster carer. This young person, their family and social worker can all be involved in considering the choice of placement. This does not have to be an either/or choice. If everyone agreed, the kinship carer and the stranger foster carer could share, for a time, caring for the young person, helping the carers to learn and support each other to manage the young person's needs.

There is developing research evidence to suggest that kinship and residence order care is equally as good as, and may be better than stranger foster care. In the face of this evidence and the other points presented in this chapter, it is to be hoped that there will be a positive shift in social services departments' attitudes to, and support for kinship care arrangements.

7

ATTACHMENT THEORY AND CHILDREN'S RIGHTS

Penelope Welbourne

Policy and practice relating to children is subject to a range of influences, which include the politics of intervention in the family, the availability of resources for intervention, and the dominant cultural view of children and childhood (Stainton Rogers, 2001).

The specific construction of 'childhood', and of the related concept of parenting used by social workers, has profound implications for decision making in respect of children. Stainton Rogers supports the view first expressed by Parton (1985, 1997) that child protection is a 'moral and political endeavour'. Recent concern on the part of the UK government (Performance and Innovation Unit, 2000) about the functioning of the adoption service leaves little room for doubt that adoption is currently a political as well as a moral enterprise. It may be argued that the moral, political and professional issues involved in adoption are likely to be at least as complex as those in child protection decision making. This contribution aims to identify and comment on a few of the many elements that contribute to this process

The way in which children are viewed is critical to how their care is planned for. Whether they are seen as resilient or easily subject to irreparable damage, as capable or incapable, or as having rights which are primarily rights to care and protection versus being holders of rights which reflect more closely the range of adult rights, all affect the planning processes for children. This may happen as part of a conscious process of thought about the child's best interests, or as a part-perceived or ill thought through undercurrent in the decision making process.

From the 1970s onwards, theorising about the enduring effects of child–parent relationships has been a potent factor in shaping social policy for children and families. Emphasis on an uninterrupted maternal relationship influenced thinking about desirable patterns of child care in the general population as well as in local authorities and voluntary adoption agencies. The pioneering work of Bowlby (1951) focused attention on developmental aspects of child welfare needs and introduced the idea of early attachment as a key determinant of the success of parenting. A restrictive interpretation of Bowlby's early work led to a belief that children who could not be brought up by their birth parent(s) needed to be permanently placed with adoptive parents by the age of two years, if the children were to be able to form an attachment to their new parents. The implication of this narrow interpretation was that older children were assigned to other forms of long term care, frequently institutional care.

Michael Rutter says that

> early accounts emphasised the need for selective attachments to develop during a relatively brief 'sensitivity period' during the first two years of life, with the implication that even very good parenting that is provided after this watershed is too late. In keeping with the changes that have taken place in thinking about sensitive periods more generally, it has become clear that this all or nothing view required modification. There is a sensitive period during which it is highly desirable that selective attachments develop but the time frame is probably somewhat broader than initially envisaged and the effects are not as fixed and irreversible as once thought.
>
> (Rutter, 1995: 551)

Another strand of research and theory centred on the work of Clarke and Clarke (1976), who presented the case for optimism in planning for children who had experienced abuse and neglect. Their thesis was largely based on studies that demonstrated the extraordinary resilience displayed by some children with early histories of extreme deprivation. The tension between these two academic viewpoints, with their very different implications for placement policy, has moderated over time, largely because of increasing moderation in the claims made about the overarching significance of the earliest years for long-term developmental outcomes.

In 1988, Bowlby in a move away from the 'critical periods' theory, wrote that, 'a theory of developmental pathways should replace theories that involve specific phases of development' (Bowlby, 1988: 1). The initial model of attachment that incorporated the idea of 'critical periods' has now been largely abandoned. The Clarkes' thesis is that

> the life path is not predetermined by the experiences of the early years alone, but results from the long-term cumulative development of genetic and environmental interactions and transactions. This knowledge should begin to inform social policies. For example, of 34,000 children in continuous care in this country in 1995, almost half had been abused or neglected or considered to be at risk of abuse

or neglect. . . . Growing up in care is likely to reinforce early damage and make it likely that these children, without *strong* intervention [authors' italics] via fostering or adoption (in spite of the difficulties), will continue their probably doomed life path.

(Clarke and Clarke, 2000: 103)

This is a statement that broadly accords with the philosophy of current government policy on permanency: local authority care has been demonstrated to fail as a system for providing adequate reparative care for children who have experienced trauma and neglect, and presents risk factors which appear resistant to local authority attempts to control them. Whatever the difficulties associated with adoption in some circumstances, particularly late adoption and adoption of children with particularly severe histories of abuse and neglect, the evidence that adoption can work for some such children means that every planning decision for every child should be made in the understanding that rates and statistics are inadequate predictors of individual outcomes.

Similarly, the optimism of the 1970s that 'no child is unadoptable' may have incorporated a naïve confidence in the abilities of adoptive parents to provide compensatory input beyond reasonable expectations. The increase in breakdown rates for adoptive placements from the late 1980s suggests that more risks were taken in arranging placements and this was reflected in the failure rate, compared with the rate during the early days of the permanency movement. There is now greater caution about placing children over the age of nine who have been badly damaged psychologically by abuse. Research has consistently shown that children under the age of about nine are likely to have better outcomes in terms of low breakdown rates than older children (Triseliotis *et al.*, 1997: 44). History prior to placement is a potential risk factor: parental rejection, abuse or deprivation prior to placement has been found to be independently associated with placement breakdown (Thoburn, 1995; Rushton *et al.*, 2000).

An early history of neglect and abuse may cause lasting physiological damage as well as behavioural changes for young children, with implications for both early and late adoption (Glaser, 2000). With older children, early attachment difficulties are likely to have been compounded by other adversities, including changes of carer and longer exposure to neglect or abuse. There may be a higher level of problem behaviours (but not anxiety or depression) among later adopted children compared with those adopted earlier, although many late adoptions are successful, even if they may be more stressful for adopters and adopted children than early adoptions (Haugaard *et al.*, 1999). Placements made in middle and late childhood do have a good chance of being successful. Perhaps three out of every four 'late' placements may become stable within the first year, with prior experience of rejection a possible risk factor for early placement breakdown (Rushton *et al.*, 2000).

In the longer-term, some of these placements do fail, but it may be that better selection and preparation of children and adopters, coupled with better quality support post-adoption could ameliorate this.

The interplay of individual characteristics, physiological responses and behavioural/cognitive adaptation to adversity is so complex that no one existing theory is able to address all the processes involved in recovery, much less predict outcomes other than in very general terms. Viewing children as individuals with the potential to display resilience as well as attract risk factors is a positive development in planning for children after the hegemony of early attachment theory and the over-optimism of the early permanency movement.

In 1999, under 10 per cent of children adopted were under one-year-old at adoption, but more than 40 per cent of adopted children were first 'admitted to care' by the age of six months (DoH, 1999; Ivaldi, 1998). The delay which occurs once adoption has been identified as the best or least detrimental option for the child is therefore significant in the impact it may have on the child's chances of having a good experience of adoptive parenting. Murch *et al.* (1993) found that the older the child, the longer the delay associated with the legal process. Parents of older children were more likely to oppose adoption. They make the point that it is important to differentiate between proceeding at a pace appropriate for the child, which may involve proceeding more slowly on occasions, and avoidable delay.

The increasing length of court cases is a matter of concern (Beckett, 2000). The great majority of cases end up with the requested public law or adoption order being made. Only about 1 per cent of welfare recommendations made are refused by the courts, so the reason for the delay seems to be something other than the resolution of a genuinely 'winnable' contest by the parents.

Murch *et al.* (1993) note the very high proportion of adoption cases going to court in which an adoption order is made, even in contested cases. In this study, only two of 1,268 cases were refused adoption orders. The apparent 'official' consensus about the child's best interests raises the question as to whether adoption agencies only present 'low risk' cases to the courts. Alternatively, are the courts overly ready to accept the local authority view that rehabilitation is impossible and adoption is in the child's best interests?

If the increase in the number of adoptions proposed by the government following the Prime ministerial review and the subsequent Adoption and Children Bill materialises, it will be interesting to see whether the inclusion of a larger number of children in the adoption process means that more cases are contested more closely. Court cases could become even longer, or more applications might be refused by the courts. Pressure to reduce the time-scale of court cases will put pressure on local authorities to demonstrate to the court's satisfaction that rehabilitation with the child's birth family is not a safe or reasonable option. This has implications for practice and for parents' rights if the 'window of opportunity' for them to present their case becomes smaller.

Children's rights in adoption are problematic, and the extent to which children are seen as having rights and the kind of rights they are considered to have depends on the prevailing philosophy of adoption agencies. Most principles are shared, crucially that children's best interests are undoubtedly best promoted by good quality consistent parenting such as that provided in a stable caring family with 'psychological parents' who may or may not be biologically related to the child. However, principles are one thing, and the interpretation of those principles quite another.

In adoption, decisions are made more complex by the child's history of attachment to other previous carers, which may include foster carers and extended family members. Firstly, most adopted children will have been attached to their biological parents. They may have been securely or insecurely attached, but they will have been attached nevertheless, to a greater or lesser degree. A dominant ideology in adoption in the 1980s, now seen as unrealistic, was the 'total severance model', in which children were expected to sever their attachments to their birth parents in order to clear the way for attachment to new parents (Thoburn, 1996: 131). Many children who have been abused show a behavioural pattern of attachment to their main carer consistent with secure attachment to their carers. 'Use of this (traditional) category system, however, led to a surprisingly large number of maltreated infants being classified as secure, a finding that contradicts expectations arising from attachment theory' (Pipp-Seigal *et al.*, 1999: 25). Other behavioural indices relating to the child's behaviour have been used to extend the classification schema, but such practice is potentially controversial (Vondra and Barnett, 1999: 17). Not all children who are placed for adoption will have been neglected or ill-treated for a prolonged period. An example is a parental mental health crisis which may be resolved but which may develop into a long-term problem: a pattern of 'good enough' care for a child may then deteriorate below an acceptable standard with limited hope of recovery. The child's early relationship with the birth parents may have been secure and positive. Given that the proportion of children in the general population who do not test as 'securely attached' is in the region of 40 per cent, it is 'not sensible to regard 40 per cent of infants as showing biologically abnormal development. . . . The category of insecure attachment cannot be equated with psychopathology or disorder' (Rutter, 1995: 559).

Neither assumptions about the quality of children's early attachments or presumed dysfunction of the majority of adopted children's early attachments could be used to justify the practice of severance of contact on adoption. The question remains how much emphasis should be placed on the preservation of family links, both those that involve attachment and those that do not, in the promotion of the child's future welfare.

Attempts to bridge the gap in the child's knowledge and understanding of their history using techniques such as life story work may not be as helpful to the child as might be hoped. The positive effect of direct work with children pre-placement has been shown to have limited impact (Rushton *et al.*, 1997/8). This may be because the work was not always thorough or skilled enough to make a difference in the context of children's life events that may have been too overwhelming to be responsive to the level of input available.

In decisions about contact made under the Children Act 1989, it is the child's interest that determines whether or not and how contact should occur. It will be interesting to see whether inclusion of the principle that the child's welfare should be the paramount consideration in adoption cases has an impact on decisions about continuing contact between adopted children and their biological families. There is evidence that contact between birth families and adopted children does not undermine placements, as was feared, and may actually promote successful outcomes in adoption (Ryburn, 1996; Adcock *et al.*, 1993). Fratter *et al.* (1991) found that contact with birth families had no adverse effect on attachment to the new family, even with children placed early, before the age of seven. Fratter also found that adoptive parents were ultimately positive about the effects of continuing contact, even in cases in which the adoption had been contested by birth parents.

Children's rights are beginning to develop more rapidly after years of discussion about the kind of rights children may actually enjoy (Fortin, 1999). Britain is a signatory to the UN Convention on the Rights of the Child (1989). Article 8(1) states that, 'Parties undertake to respect the rights of the child to preserve his or her identity, including nationality, name and family relations as recognised by law without unlawful interference' and 'when the child is unlawfully deprived of some or all of the elements of his or her identity, the state has a duty to take steps aimed at speedily re-establishing his or her identity' (Article 8(2)).

Adoption appears to be excluded from the provisions of Article 8 because it is a lawful 'deprivation of identity'. The extent to which identity as defined in Article 8 is lost varies from one adopted child to another, but some such loss is inevitable. One might question the great divide between children's Article 8 rights when deprived of their identity by agents or influences other than the state acting within the law, and adoption, which for many years under the 'severance model' represented a legal extinction of prior identity. The broad and aspirational framing of much of the Convention on the Rights of the Child means that it is unclear whether children do have rights under Article 8 when subject to extinction of parental rights in adoption cases. It would however seem reasonable to question why extinction of birth parents' parental rights should entail a loss on the part of the child of the right to respect for other aspects of identity which would not jeopardise the child's safety or future development, such as protection of sibling and other family relationships. When one considers the over-representation of children whose culture is not that of the dominant white UK population in the 'care' population (Barn, 1993) and the moral, professional and political issues associated with this, the applicability of a child's right to preservation of identity is a significant issue:

> with the great majority of adoptions by non-kin in Britain now involving older children, the emphasis has shifted from disclosure to managing openness and contact. . . . Revealing adoption, assisted reproduction or the reality of status of other separated children . . . should not have been a scientific but a moral issue. Nevertheless, the studies . . . have shown that being truthful and honest with children about their status, circumstances, roots, genealogy and general background is central to their identity formation and their mental health.
> (Treacher and Katz, 2000: 84)

Thoburn (1995) argues that it was responsiveness to the needs of adopters that motivated the 'clean break' approach to adoption. The supporting theory was that severing the child's early, possibly damaging attachment to the biological parent/s would free the child to develop new, healthier attachments in the new family. Life story work developed as a way of facilitating the process. Older children who did not wish to lose contact with birth parents and were able to articulate their wishes were frequently not listened to by social workers. In retrospect, the idea that severing an attachment against the expressed wishes of a child would promote and enable the development of new secure attachments seems surprising, and only tenable in an adult-centred view of adoption. However, a developing sense of the importance of respecting established relationships is in the process of becoming embedded in permanent placement practice.

Siblings present a particular challenge to placement practice. Siblings may represent a source of support and security, or have acquired a caring role that cannot easily be relinquished, having possibly been acquired as a result of a prolonged period of adversity. However, 'in adoption planning, Ellison found that virtually two-thirds of the children in her study who were to be adopted were separated from some or all of their looked after siblings, and almost half of these were placed apart from all their siblings . . . two-thirds of those with siblings were placed without any of them and, where they were with siblings, this was typically because they had come into placement together rather than because of active planning' (Mullender, 2000: 323). Mullender concludes 'perhaps . . . we need to recognise more fully that it is wrong for adoption to cut people off from their roots'.

Adoption has been susceptible to varying conceptualisations of childhood, from a state of passive receipt of care, to an emerging view of children as people with rights that extend beyond fundamental needs for nurture and 'psychological parenting'. In the past, children have been the subject of policies which were aimed at returning them to an emotional 'tabula rasa' in order to facilitate the (adult) purposes of adoption. More recently, they have begun to be seen as individuals with a history which is a part of their identity and which should be protected by right.

In 1926 in the case of Thain the judge explained his decision to return a seven-year-old child to her father's care after six years in foster care on the basis of the child's presumed adaptability. She would be 'greatly distressed and upset', but 'at her tender age, one knows from experience how mercifully transient are the effects of partings and other sorrows, and how soon the novelty of fresh surroundings and new associations effaces the recollection of former days and kind friends' (cited in Bainham, 1998: 11).

The adult centred view of young children as incapable of deep or prolonged sorrow is mercifully no longer a prevalent view in care planning. Ideas about risk, need, vulnerability and resilience all have a part to play in a child centred service, together with respect for children as rights holders. Recent developments in understanding children's perceptual and recall abilities have established that with appropriate support children can communicate about past events and their wishes and feelings with a clarity and reliability comparable to that of adults (Spencer and Flynn, 1990). They are capable of making complex decisions about their future welfare even in circumstances that may present adults with extreme difficulty, and say which decisions they want adults to make for them (Alderson, 1998). There is no longer any valid excuse for treating children as 'objects of concern' (Butler-Sloss, 1988: 245).

There is congruence between the messages from research about the needs of children who cannot be brought up by their birth parents, and developments in thinking about children as rights holders. Both indicate the need for child care and legal systems which respond early and purposefully when children are abused or neglected, and which are capable of responding to the child as a holder of individual rights. In adoption, this means respecting childrens' future need for integration and coherence in developing their identity as well as meeting their current needs for care and nurture.

References

Adcock, M., Kaniuk, J. and White, R. (1993), *Exploring openness in adoption*, Croydon, Significant Publications.

Alderson, P. (1993), *Children's consent to surgery*, Buckingham, Open University Press.

Bainham, A. (1998), *Children: the modern law* (second edition), Bristol, Family Law.

Barn, R. (1993), *Black children in the public care system*, London, Batsford.

Beckett, C. (2000), Waiting for court decisions: a kind of limbo, *Adoption and Fostering*, 24(2): 55.

Bowlby, J. (1951), *Maternal care and mental health*, Geneva, World Health Organisation.

Bowlby, J. (1988), Developmental psychology comes of age, *American Journal of Psychiatry*, 145: 1–10.

Butler-Sloss, E. (1998), *Report of the enquiry into child abuse in Cleveland 1987*, Cmnd 412, London, HMSO.

Clarke, A. and Clarke, A. (1976), *Early experience: myth and evidence*, London, Open Books.

Clarke, A. and Clarke, A. (2000), *Early experience and the life path*, London, Jessica Kingsley.

Department of Health (1999), *Children looked after by local authorities*, London, Department of Health.

Fortin, J. (1998), *Children's rights and the developing law*, London, Butterworths.

Fratter, J., Rowe, J., Sapsford, D. and Thoburn, J. (1991), *Permanent family placement: a decade of experience*, London, BAAF.

Glaser, D. (2000), Child abuse and neglect and the brain: a review, *Journal of Child Psychology and Psychiatry*, 41(1): 97.

Haugaard, J., Wojslawowicz, J. and Palmer, M. (1999), Outcomes in adolescent and older-child adoptions, *Adoption Quarterly*, 3(1): 61.

Howe, D. (ed.) (1996), *Attachment and loss in child and family social work*, Hants, Ashgate.

Ivaldi, G. (1998), *Children adopted from care: an examination of agency adoptions in England, 1996*, London, British Agencies for Adoption and Fostering.

Mullender, A. (ed.) (1999), *We are family: sibling relationships in permanent family placement and beyond*, London, British Agencies for Adoption and Fostering.

Murch, M., Lowe, N., Borkowski, M., Copner, R. and Griew, K. (1993), *Pathways to adoption research project*, London, HMSO.

Parton, N. (1985), *The politics of child abuse*, Basingstoke, Macmillan.

Performance and Innovation Unit (2000), *Review on adoption: issues for consultation*, London, Cabinet Office.

Pipp-Seigal, S., Seigal, C. and Dean, J. (1999), Neurological aspects of the disorganised/disoriented attachment classification system, in Vondra, J. and Barnett, D. (eds) *Atypical attachment in infancy and early childhood among children at developmental risk*, Oxford, Blackwell.

Rushton, A., Quinton, D., Dance, C. and Mayes, D. (1997), Preparation for permanent placement: evaluating direct work with older children, *Adoption and Fostering*, 21: 41.

Rushton, A., Dance, C. and Quinton, D. (1997/1998), Findings from a UK-based study of late permanent placements, *Adoption Quarterly*, 3(3): 51.

Rutter, M. (1995), Clinical implications of attachment concepts: retrospect and prospect, *Journal of Child Psychology and Psychiatry*, 36(4): 549.

Ryburn, M. (1994), *Open adoption: research, theory and practice*, Aldershot, Avebury.

Ryburn, M. (1996), A study of post-adoption contact in compulsory adoptions, *British Journal of Social Work*, 27.

Spencer, J. R. and Flynn, R. (1990), *The evidence of children: the law and the psychology*, London, Blackstone.

Stainton Rogers, W. (2001), Constructing childhood, constructing child concern, in Foley, P., Roche, J. and Tucker, S. (eds) *Children in society: contempory theory, policy and practice*, Basingstoke, Palgrave.

Thoburn, J. (1996), Psychological parenting and child placement: 'But we want to have our cake and eat it,' in D. Howe (ed.) *Attachment and loss in child and family social work*, Aldershot, Ashgate.

Treacher, A. and Katz, I. (eds) (2000), *The dynamics of adoption: social and personal perspective*, London, Jessica Kingsley Publishers.

Triseliotis, J., Shireman, J. and Hundleby, M. (1997), *Adoption theory, policy and practice*, London, Cassell.

Vondra, J. and Barnett, D. (1999), *Atypical attachment in infancy and early childhood among children at developmental risk*, Oxford, Blackwell.

8

'I'LL TAKE HER IN'

Chris Purnell

My mother, Daisy, was born in Scarborough in July 1911 to an unmarried woman. The twin effects of grinding poverty and social stigma drove her to desperation. Unlike many women at that time, my grandmother rejected the options of abandonment or infanticide, usually by smothering. Instead, she looked for a home for my mother and the manner in which she did this was quite extraordinary. She took my mother in her arms and knocked on doors in her neighbourhood until she found someone who would accept her into their family. This was a form of care where a seemingly callous action was actually in a crude way compassionate. At least she had some knowledge of the person who was going to care for the infant.

The woman who accepted her was, seemingly, the antithesis of the good adoptive parent. Annie Morris was 51 years old at a time when life expectancy was 50. She was a washer woman living in a single room. Her occupation meant that room was used for both washing and drying. The drying was done from ceiling racks and this made the entire room permanently wet. She lived in poverty with most weeks ending either with no food or an increase in 'tick' at the local shop. The room was shared with mice. Her own children were adults and her principal motivation in taking in my mother was to have company. My mother was to be looked after in return for being an ever present companion.

When Daisy was old enough to go to school the bond of reliance that had grown between mother and daughter meant that the experience was traumatic for them both.

Since my mother had been handed to Mrs Morris as a chance offering, they had not been separated. School laws determined that they had to be. This challenge threw up a conflict between the law and my gran-ma's needs. This was compounded by the usual reservations and doubts that many working class people had at that time about the value of education for girls.

Mother and daughter conspired to agree on how many odd days at home could be safely taken off without the interference of officialdom. This was important as they were both deeply aware that the authorities could put their living arrangements in jeopardy. The dreaded worst possibility was that her biological mother might reappear and reclaim my mother. In the end, Daisy took one or two days off each week which satisfied both the authorities and mother and daughter. As a very intelligent person, this lack of formal education was to cast a long shadow.

When my mother was 24 she married Walter, a joiner also from Scarborough, and in the following year they moved to Leeds. This was in the depths of the Depression with cut-throat competition for skilled jobs. In an intensely political era the only thing that mattered in my mother's eyes was the family. Politics, religion, or any ideology were so much rubbish if they interfered with the unity of the family. They were both devoted to their family and the legacy of economic instability in the 1930s meant that some very cautious decisions were made. He was involved in Directed Labour in the war effort and worked exceptionally long hours, building bombers. All the additional money went to buying a house. Those long hours gave him a massive wage which he used to pay off the house. For different reasons, Walter and Daisy needed the stability which debt free property ownership gave them.

Annie was 76 when they left Scarborough to look for work and economic stability. It was quite clear that she needed help but her pathological fear of the workhouse meant she would not accept any official help. This meant that there was only one condition to my parents' marriage: that Annie would be cared for and kept in the family home for as long as was necessary. The newly married couple shared their two bedroom house with her for ten years. As the family grew with my sisters born in 1936 and 1941 respectively, living conditions became difficult. But my mother had been taken in by a woman who had one room and one bed and she hadn't flinched, so 'what was good for the goose was good for the gander' as she used to say.

Annie wasn't an easy woman to live with and old age was making her more decrepit. Being frightened of electricity where she firmly believed that it leaked, like gas, was only one of her quirks; thinking that indoor toilets were unhygienic was also hard for my father to accept. Annie's bossing of my mother and her girls was also a source of enormous tension. That coupled with the war years made life very demanding. However everything has to be placed in a context. They felt that they were laying really firm foundations for themselves and their family: and they were.

When I was born in 1945 my parents both finally agreed that living conditions had became impossible. With three children to be cared for and the fact that Annie was now 86 meant that her care had to be formalised. The incoming Labour Government finally laid to rest the vile means-testing era of the 1930s and the legacy of the workhouse. And so she accepted that the world had truly changed for the better and it wasn't a trick. She left our house to move into residential care. Meanwhile, Daisy's family were benefiting from the enhanced education provision as eventually two of her children went to university and took professional jobs. My other sister in her turn adopted a boy who is now a French polisher. Daisy's legacy of care and love continues today.

Annie died in 1951 aged 90 years old having led a long life which spanned different worlds. From Queen Victoria's heyday and the height of Imperial Britain to a Labour Government – what an amazing story. My mother died in Otley in 2000 at the age of 88. She emerged from an act which looked on the surface like an act of utter barbarity to being hugely successful in her creation of a stable family. Both women were ordinary people who met life's challenges head-on, fending for themselves with a very pre-Welfare State mentality.

This adoptive experience was rich with an unequivocal and reciprocated love. As my mother used to say: 'The woman who brings you up is your mother'.

Part II

THE EXPERIENCE OF BIRTH PARENTS

INTRODUCTION

Until comparatively recently birth parents have been the obscured side of the adoption triangle. Adoption is an attempt to secure a better future for a child and the emphasis has been on the child's integration into its new family and support for the adoptive parents. There has always (rightly) been enormous stress on the emotional needs of the child and the task which faces the adoptive parent. This has meant, in practice, that the birth parent has been someone left behind after the adoption order has been made, with an implication that her – for it usually is a 'her' – needs do not exist. That she will most likely make new relationships, have more children and may need support during the interim period, is usually ignored.

As we state elsewhere in this book, it is not so long ago that adoption meant a surgical removal of the child from its birth family with the consequent severance allowing little possibility of contact between child and birth family. Arguments were made for not telling the child that they were adopted because the information would be harmful (Ansfield, 1971) or would complicate the adoption. While unlike an earlier time when 'adopted children were often not informed of their status and could be traumatized to discover it by accident' (Department of Health, 1993), adopted children were sometimes told in the 1950s. However, the myth that they would not need to seek their birth parents if they were happily adopted was perpetuated by the fact that adoptees in England and Wales could not secure information to search for their birth parents prior to the Children Act 1975. Section 36, the relevant part of the legislation, later came to form Section 51 of the Adoption Act 1976. (Scotland had had that right since 1930; adopted people in Northern Ireland gained it in 1989.) The relationship between birth parent and birth child was marked by a mutual lack of knowledge about each other.

But when adopted people obtained the right to search for their birth parent, the secondary position of birth parents was typified by the fact that no corresponding right was granted to the birth parent and this remains the case in the UK, although in some other countries, like, for example, Australia and New Zealand, this is not the case.

75

Such a right for birth parents to be able to search for their adult child, while agitated for by professionals in the UK, has never got itself onto the political agenda. It did not feature on the Blair government's list of reforms that led to the Adoption and Children Act 2002. This is further evidence of the snowpaking of birth parents from the history books.

For over a decade, adoption professionals and a lobby of birth mothers have been campaigning for intermediary services to facilitate contact between a searching birth parent and child or to let an adopted person know of an inquiry and interest being registered. Whilst the national Adoption Contact Register was set up in 1991, it has a low profile and matchings have been few.

If we move from the analogy of adoption triangle to adoption circle – an analogy more in keeping with the tenor of much present day adoption practice and philosophy – birth parents, as much as their adopted children, have a need to square the circle (Feast *et al.*, 1998). They feel the need to ask questions, to satisfy themselves. Is their child happy? Is he or she safe and well? Does the child feel that adoption was a rejection? Or that it was not loved? Does the child feel that the birth parent's decision was justified? Does the child know that it has never been forgotten by its birth parent? And when birth parents do try and find their adopted adult children – as some do and can through the intermediary services which do exist and are offered by adoption agencies, like, for example, the Children's Society – or when they are sought, they want to tell their child why they were adopted and that their being placed for adoption did not mean that they were not loved. We know that many birth parents want information at some time during their lives (Hughes and Logan, 1993).

The feelings of both child and birth mother and the experience of reunion are given in the following pages. In chapter 9, a birth mother, Audrey, and her daughter Aline, tell the story of losing a son, finding him again, and for Aline, finding a brother she suspected all along she had. Christopher Hignett describes how in his mid-fifties, his mother sought him out and the rewards that brought. In chapter 11, an adoptive mother and social work lecturer writes a powerful letter to an anonymous social worker, describing poetically the needs of birth mothers everywhere.

Just as adoption has been remade over the years, that has also involved the remaking or redefining of the birth parent – from natural parent to first parent to (now) birth parent. Such changes in nomenclature reflect changing attitudes so that we now recognise that the birth parent, too, needs to be considered not only for her own sake but also for the sake of the child's own sense of identity. As Simmonds (2002) says of the compounding of telling children the truth, of granting them the right to search and the institution of open adoption:

> All these ideas are aimed at providing adults and children with access to a narrative that is in varying degrees psychologically and socially sound and is a satisfying response to the problem of curiosity.

Simmonds does not say as much but it must be stressed that the 'adults' in that statement are not only adopted adults but birth parents, too: they require access to a narrative; they, too, need to feel a completeness which comes from knowledge of who their child has become and how they stand in relation to them.

Professor John Triseliotis and colleagues asked 99 birth mothers how they felt on hearing that their adopted adult son or daughter had wanted to have contact with them. The reactions were 'pleased' (50), 'excited, happy' (55), 'surprised' (20). Only two said that they were 'nervous, worried' and the same number were 'worried' and 'frightened'. When 100 mothers were asked if contact had been a positive experience, 67 said 'very positive', 27 'positive' and six were not sure (Triseliotis, 2001).

While reference in this chapter is often to birth parents some matters, but definitely not all, apply to birth fathers. However, it the case that the term birth parent means, practically and usefully, birth mother. Some birth fathers do seek their child, but not many, and only a minority of birth children seek their father. One significant reason is that often that adopted people have less information about their fathers. For example, he is rarely named on the birth certificate. Often he does not become 'real' until the adopted person has received information from the adoption records. The adopted person may also feel unable to contact the birth father if the birth mother feels unhappy about it.

Feast and Howe (2000) found that 75 per cent of those in their study sought their birth mother and only 38 per cent their birth father. What the authors refer to as the most ambitious group was the 11 per cent who hoped to find both birth parents and birth siblings. But once the search was underway, 91 per cent of searchers decided to look first for their birth mother. Sachdev (1993) found few adopted people who wanted to look for their birth father; indeed, only 20 per cent said that they ever thought about him.

When it comes to searching, there are some parallel feelings which adopted people and birth parents exhibit. For example, some adopted people do not search for fear of rejection, yet rejection is also a fear that is held by birth parents. As Barbara, a birth mother, said:

> I would dearly love to find my son who was adopted 30 years ago but I am now scared in case he doesn't want to hear from me. Maybe he is resentful so it's easier for me to live with fantasy rather than the reality of rejection.
>
> (Barbara, 2002)

While the memory of an adopted child is never lost to the birth mother, the adoption may well have been thirty or more years ago. Since then she may have married someone who is not the father of the child and have had another family who do not know about the adoption. In a few cases birth mothers do not want to re-establish that link that was once severed. 'Angie' (Feast *et al.*,

1998) experienced perhaps an extreme reaction from her birth mother when she traced her: 'As far as I am concerned she is not my daughter.' That first birth – the half-brother or sister of the children of the second relationship – may well be a secret not even known to the new partner. Fear of rejection in such cases may not just be that of adopted child toward birth parent but rejection by the new family – particularly the children who may fear that they will be displaced by the new, older half-brother or sister. If a birth parent chooses not to try and find what has happened to their adopted adult child it may be that not having told her husband and children, she has no wish to go back. Or the rejection may stem from the pain of having a lost past, a lost opportunity to have brought up the child.

For birth mothers the sense of loss, grief and guilt felt by giving up her child, or by having had her child taken away from her, can be overwhelming. Relinquishing, as it is called, whatever the circumstances, has a lasting and often life-long impact. Many birth parents, even when involved in subsequent relationships and after they have had other children, secretly remember the child they lost, especially on key anniversaries like birthdays. One birth mother told one of the editors of this volume: 'What if your child dies and you don't know anything about it? You wouldn't even be able to go to the funeral'. After a twelve-year search, another mother found that her daughter died when she was eleven – 'All the dreams and hopes I had created over the years had to be rebuilt, while I came to terms with her death and the realisation that I will never meet her again' (quoted in Feast, 2002). On the farewell visit to her five-year-old child, another birth mother with mild learning difficulties, told a social worker that she wasn't opposing the adoption (she had not protected her daughter from sexual abuse), and that she planned to open a bank account for her daughter and work herself to death. When mothers do give their children up, it is often a courageous and moving decision made in the genuine belief they are doing the best for their child.

This loss, grief and guilt may have long-term and very injurious effects on the birth mother's mental and emotional well-being. Several studies (Bouchier et al., 1991; Howe et al., 1992; Wells, 1993; Hughes and Logan, 1993) have shown that the loss of a child through adoption may profoundly affect the birth mother's mental health and damage her ability to cope. These repercussions may last all the mother's life. Howe and Feast (2000) report that

> it is now believed by many counsellors and support workers that the high incidence of emotional and physical disorders described by birth mothers is likely to be the result of repressed mourning and the consequences of living with the unresolved losses and traumas associated with their child's adoption.

In 1998 the Post-Adoption Action Group mounted a successful conference 'Balancing the equation', and since then annual 'services of hope, thanksgiving and reconciliation' for people affected by adoption have been held on each Mothering Sunday.

There are halfway houses to reach in seeking assurance about the consequences of that long-ago decision to allow adoption. Some people – and this may apply also to the adopted person – do not want a meeting. The birth mother may only be prepared to let the child she placed for adoption know that she is alive and well and to offer any information which may be required. Equally, the adopted person may simply wish to let the birth parent know that they are alright and happy and healthy. But we do know that 90 per cent of non-searching adopted people who were informed of a birth mother's enquiry went on to have some form of contact. We also know that only 7 per cent of birth mothers refused to have any contact with their adopted adult child (Howe and Feast, 2000).

But even if a meeting is desired, we know that even when a birth parent is found, it does not automatically lead to a long-term relationship (Howe and Feast, 2000; Sachdev, 1998). The past cannot be reconstructed or lived over again. One or only a few meetings may be enough – facts are obtained, curiosity is satisfied. (Of course, the long-term effects of finding may well be disproportionate to the length of time of any contact no matter how brief.) In Sachdev's 1992 study, he found that only 51 per cent of searchers had continued contact with their birth mother although 97 per cent of adopted people had no regrets about searching. In the same study, Sachdev found that 17 per cent of adopted people ended their relationship with their mother after the first meeting. Could this be related to the same author's 1988 finding that only 19.8 per cent of adopted people characterised the new-found relationship as one of that of mother and child, while the remaining 73.2 per cent described it as a friendship or said that their birth mother felt like an acquaintance? But Howe and Feast (2000) report that 63 per cent of searchers and 55 per cent of non-searchers were still in touch with their birth mothers five years after the first contact.

All of these issues are comparatively modern ones, occasioned by the possibilities arising from the provisions of the Children Act 1975. But the Children Act 1989 brought birth parents into the possibility of closer and sharper relationships with their children from the time of adoption, rather than many years later, through open adoption. This now means that an increasing number of adopted children have some contact with their birth parent or parents.

In addition to the emotional needs which birth parents can feel about a child adopted many years ago and referred to above, open adoption, which is part and parcel of the adoption from the very beginning, can increase the acceptance of the adoption, however mixed the feelings are. So far as adoptive parents are concerned, open adoption may overcome some of the fears and problems, already mentioned, which can be experienced later in life in the event of a successful search by their child or their child's birth parent.

Contact can reduce adoptive parents fear of the birth parents; reduce their fantasy of how attached the child is to their birth parent; lead to a greater understanding of the child; and reinforce the adoption.

Open adoption also recognises, as Greenwood (2000) states, the complexity of human relations; that is, that we never let go, we never forget, we carry our past with us always even if, at times, we do not or cannot acknowledge it. Greenwood is herself an expert witness – her own daughter was adopted and so was her grandson. She is a psychologist and has three other daughters. Touching on another aspect of the adoptive parent–birth parent axis, she claims that her daughter's experience (with the grandson) was undermined by professionals who could not accept that there were two 'good' mothers. It is an unfortunate side effect of – or perhaps a supposed justification for – the sidelining of the birth mother that she needs to be seen as 'bad' or at very least deficient. When the mother is unmarried, she is, as Greenwood states, seen as representing sexuality for pleasure and is supposed to be outside of control, though this may not be the case. Teenager mothers are too often seen as stupid, feckless, irresponsible, even queue-jumpers of the local authority housing waiting list.

Such attitudes to unmarried mothers were epitomised in the policies of the last Conservative government and have found their way through to some statements by members of the Blair government. For example, Jack Straw, when Home Secretary, said that such irresponsible young women should give up their children for adoption, echoing previous remarks made a few years before by the right-wing Conservative minister, John Redwood. The idea that children are transferable packages, whose departure from the birth mother to the adoptive mother is not about loss, grief and human tragedy but the 'solution' of a social problem (children in the care of 'bad' mothers when so many 'good' would-be adopted parents want to take them in) indicates how irresponsible and ignorant politicians can be when populism supplants policymaking.

What we have said about birth parents' need for contact and their being able to trace their adopted adult child applies to most birth parents but cannot apply to all. There will be those who will reject such contact or who would not wish to exercise their right to search if it were legislated for (just as some adopted people choose not to do). The kind of contact that comes from open adoption is dependent on the maturity of the birth parents and their acknowledgement that there are two sets of parents (Prynne, 2000), as well as the willingness of adoptive parents

It is the case that for many adopted people, however happy they may be to make contact and to maintain a relationship, their real parent will always be the person who raised them. These, though, are details, albeit important ones, about the significance we accord to birth parents. Such details complicate many aspects of adoption and those who form the circle. But they cannot obscure the needs and rights of birth parents and the devastating emotional impact that comes in the train of the loss of a child through adoption.

References

Ansfield, J. (1971), *The adopted child*, US, Thomas.

Barbara (2002), case material supplied to the authors by Julia Feast.

Bouchier, P., Lambert, L. and Triseliotis J. (1991), *Parting with a child for adoption: the mother's perspective*, London, British Agencies for Adoption and Fostering.

Department of Health (1993), *Adoption: the future*, London, HMSO.

Feast, J. (2002), Will adoption bear fruit? *Community Care*, 17–23, January, pp. 40–1.

Feast, J., Marwood, M., Seabrook, S. and Webb, E. (1998), *Preparing for reunion: experiences from the adoption circle*, London, The Children's Society, 2nd edition.

Greenwood, S. (2000), Pregnant bodies and rational parenthood, in A. Treacher and I. Katz (eds) *The dynamics of adoption: social and personal perspectives*, London, Jessica Kingsley Publishing.

Howe, D., Sawbridge, P. and Hinings, D. (1992), *Half a million women: mothers who lose their children through adoption*, London, Penguin Books.

Howe, D. and Feast, J. (2000), *Adoption, search and reunion: the long-term experience of adopted adults*, London, The Children's Society.

Hughes, B. and Logan, J. (1993), *Birth parents: the hidden dimension – an evaluation of a birth parent project*, Research report, University of Manchester.

Prynne, B. (2000), The adoption experience from a social worker's point of view, in A. Treacher and I. Katz (eds) *The dynamics of adoption: social and personal perspectives*, London, Jessica Kingsley Publishing.

Sachdev, P. (1988), *Reunions and their aftermath*, Parent Finders of Ontario.

—— (1992), Adoption, reunion and after: a study of the research process and experience of adoptees, US, *Child Welfare*.

Simmonds, J. (2000), The adoption narrative: stories that we tell and those that we can't, in A. Treacher and I. Katz (eds) *The dynamics of adoption: social and personal perspectives*, London, Jessica Kingsley Publishing.

Triseliotis, J. (2001), Memorandum, *Hansard*, 21 November, pp. 123–4.

Wells, S. (1993), Post-traumatic stress disorder in birth mothers, London, *Adoption and Fostering*, 17(2).

9

AUDREY AND ALINE'S STORY

Audrey and Aline Boundy

Audrey's story

It was 1949, I was 19, unmarried and expecting a baby. Such things didn't happen in 1949. Not in my world. My boyfriend Ivor and I had such a good relationship. We had both left school the previous year and I was working in the local council offices. Ivor had gone on to do a crammer's course for his O-Levels, which he had previously failed at school. We were very happy in each other's company and needed nobody else. Then he was called up to do his military service. It was such a blow because he was sent to the south of the country, miles away from home and our only contact was through writing letters. There were no telephones, let alone mobile phones or text messages to stay in touch. I wrote to him every day, although now I wonder what on earth I could have to say every 24 hours. I used to go to his parents' house on Saturday nights to visit his mum and dad. He would phone while I was there.

After three months, Ivor got some leave and came home. I went to meet him at Newcastle Central Station together with his brother Eric. It was like all my Christmases had come together. We were both so happy. We spent nearly all his leave together and on his last night – that was when it happened. We couldn't bear to be apart and together we created our baby, David.

The next three months went back to the same pattern. If I suspected that there was something different about me, I put it aside. When I finally realised that I might be pregnant, I wrote to him. He replied that, of course, he would stand by me. My mother took me to our GP who confirmed that I was three months pregnant. It was nearly February and I was to be the chief bridesmaid at his brother's wedding. Ivor was coming home to be best man. The wedding went off very well and later that night he walked me home. I told him again that it has been confirmed I was pregnant and again he told me that everything would be OK and that we would be married. That was before he told his parents.

I was summoned to his house the next day and from then on it all went downhill. I was made to understand that he couldn't marry me because he was only 19 (as I was) and had to have a career. Ivor had somehow myste-riously disappeared from his home while I was there, so I didn't see him. The next few days were a nightmare. When I phoned his house, he just didn't come to the phone and in desperation, I got a friend to phone him and make an arrangement to meet him. When I saw him, he told me that he couldn't marry me or his parents would cut him off without a penny. Pride made me accept this and so he was out of my life.

I went to see the local Methodist minister who, with his wife, were good friends. They suggested that I move in with them when they accepted a job near London. I gratefully agreed and for the next few months lived with them and their two children in Ruislip, Middlesex. Life went on and on July 4th I was taken to hospital where David was born. By now I was just living from day to day and enjoying looking after a little baby and being with him all the time. After two weeks in hospital, I returned to the vicarage and looked after David for the next four weeks.

In the meantime, the minister has been in touch with a lady who was in charge of adoption at the National Children's Homes, which was linked to the Methodist Church. She came to see me and told me that the couple she had in mind for the adoption were a good couple who were unable to have children of their own. They desperately wanted a baby and would look after him very well.

The vicar, his wife and I discussed this and after much heart searching, I finally agreed to have David adopted. At home, I lived only with my mother who worked as my father had died when I was six years old. I had no living grandparents, so there was no-one there who could look after a baby as I also needed to work. When David was six weeks old, I took him to the adoption lady and handed him over. I returned to the vicarage and somehow got on with my life, returning home after a while.

I tried to keep in touch by sending little presents via the adoption lady to David but after about four months of this she wrote to me and said it would be better for everyone if I could try to forget about him and let him go. I couldn't forget about him of course and each year, especially on his birthday, I remembered him and wondered how he was, what he looked like, and how he was doing. Many years later, after I had married and had two more chil-dren, I received a phone call from a work colleague of David's. He had been trying to find me and had eventually succeeded. We met and it was so unbe-lievable. He was married to a lovely girl and they had two daughters. We have kept in touch ever since.

Aline's story

It was April 1977 and Mam and I were in the dining room that morning, cleaning together. I can remember the smell of furniture polish, the gleaming, dark wood of the solid dining table and side-board, the watery spring sun coming in through the south-facing windows. The house, an old farmhouse, was set back off the main road, so the only noises which punctuated our easy conversation were the occasional chirping of birds, or bleating of sheep.

The phone rang.

Mam went to answer it. I carried on cleaning, half-listening to what she said to see if I could work out who it was. She didn't say very much. 'Yes, yes . . .' a little hesitantly, then, 'I'm sure you can't imagine how I feel'. Suddenly I felt excitement. Shivers ran down my spine. I sensed that the phone call was more than it seemed. She didn't take long and came back into the doorway as if stunned.

'What's the matter? Who was it?' I asked.

'Come in the kitchen. Let's put the kettle on and I'll tell you'.

The kitchen was a darker room, north facing but with cheery yellow floral wallpaper and bright lights. She filled the kettle, switched it on and looked at me.

'I don't know where to start' she said.

'I think I can tell you', I cut in, 'I have another brother or sister, don't I?' She stared at me. 'How do you know?'

'I don't know' I said, 'I just do'.

We had had these telepathic experiences before, my mother and I. I remember running after school into the office where she used to work when I was about 12 years old, and her asking me, as usual, what had happened at school that day.

'Not much' I shrugged my shoulders.

'Oh?' she had said, in a way that made me look at her. As I looked into her eyes, I found myself saying, 'Our Robbie's going to be Head Boy'. Robbie was my cousin, six years my senior, in his final year at school, the Upper Sixth. I had no idea that he's been chosen, or indeed that there was any selection process going on, and yet somehow my mother told me, without words. This same feeling of knowing something I hadn't been told, had come back with that phone call. But was it really telepathy? If I am truthful, there were other snippets of knowledge, ideas, which had become so vague through time that I was no longer able to tell if they were real or just childish fantasy, floating around in my head. As a small child, I loved to rummage through drawers and cupboards. Among my favourites was my dad's old wooden roll-top desk, with its leather-bound blotter and all the tiny compartments and drawers. Drawers full of keys, string, pen-knives, old pencils, strange geometrical measuring instruments (Dad was Chief Engineer and Surveyor for the local council), a monocular souvenir from the battlefields of the Second World War, an endless supply of paper and an extremely ancient Anglepoise lamp with excellent illumination. The drawers all required a different knack to open. Lift a bit then pull sharply out; go gently, it slips easily and so on.

In my mother's bedroom, I loved to look through her jewellery box; also the drawers of her dressing table, which were full of gloves, from fine cotton lace to kid-skin, to enormous furry mock leopard ones for winter. Lots of silky head-scarves. And then, in the bottom of her wardrobe, there were more bags and boxes. In one of those bags I found a diary. The hand-writing actually looked more like my aunt's than my mother's, although they wrote in a similar way. It was for 1949. There weren't many entries, but there was one which talked about going to a party and feeling very tired. The entry for the next day really caught my attention. 'Baby born'. I can remember thinking it must have been my cousin Robbie, although the dates did seem a little too long ago. I continued to leaf through and came across the only other entry in the diary, six weeks later. 'My last full day with the baby'. I was very confused. I must have been about eight or nine years old. I could sense something did not fit in with the aunt interpretation and yet my curiosity would not let me keep quiet. I asked Mam straight out, as children often do. 'Do I have another brother or sister?' She was shocked at the question and asked why I asked. I told her about the diary. She asked where I had found it. I fibbed, saying my little brother had given it to me. The next time I went to look at the diary, it had gone.

During my adolescence, the memory of this incident grew vague and indistinct. Yet a seed of curiosity had been sown, and although through time the interpretation of what had really happened and what I imagined to have happened became fuzzy and blurred, the idea of the possibility of the existence of another sibling remained.

I became interested, during my teenage years, in the whole cyclical process of becoming a woman and eventually a mother. I liked nothing better than to be told the story of my own birth; who can resist being the central character in a drama? My mam had been for yet another check-up at the local clinic that morning. 'I just wish it were here! I feel as if I've been this size forever!' she complained to her mid-wife. 'Well, I didn't tell you this' replied the nurse conspiratorially, 'but go home, drink half a bottle of cod liver oil and a glass of orange juice and wait and see'.

She trudged back home in the icy February morning, stopping at the chemist's on the way to buy the cod liver oil. She struggled up one flight of stairs to the small flat, drank her strange cocktail and quickly prepared lunch for my dad, who, regular as clockwork, walked in at 12.30, ate and returned to work. At about two o'clock, as she was just finishing clearing up the meal, her labour pains started. I was born at a quarter to five, not quite three hours later.

Some years later, I realised that this was awfully short for a first labour and I knew there was something else submerged in my memory that was linked, but at that point, they were just two separate ideas in different orbits, circling in my mind. Sometimes surfacing, reminding me separately of their existence. Occasionally, they would cross paths and I'd try to hold them captive, hoping that if I could somehow force them to reveal to me why they continued to circle around in my brain, I'd find some answers. I didn't. Until the phone call, which caught them as their paths crossed and froze them for a split second; and then I knew.

'His name is David' said Mam. 'I'd called him Richard, after my father, but his adoptive parents called him David'. She paused, then continued, eyes wet. 'I was only 19. It was very difficult. I went down to London to have him, but everybody here knew. In those days, people had a very low opinion of unmarried mothers'.

'So, what are you going to do?' I asked

'He wants me to go down to London to meet him. I think I'll go next week!'

10

LOST AND FOUND

An adopted person's story

Christopher Hignett

My parents always tried to tell me the truth about my adoption, although I perceived it differently at different times in my life and it always contained conundrums. I want to start with my 54th birthday. We are opening my cards and presents. Among them and saved to last is a large brown envelope that arrived two days previously. The address is handwritten in a script I do not immediately recognise. It could be that of any of a number of friends. Rather more intriguingly there is a message in the top left hand corner: 'This is not a circular. Not to be opened until 28th November'. Almost certainly the message is what has promoted the envelope to be the last to be opened. I do so and extract a booklet that is bound like a student dissertation and a letter. The booklet is entitled 'The Smith Family Tree', and within a few seconds of looking at the letter, my partner, who is reading it over my shoulder, says, 'You know who this is from, don't you? It's your mother'.

And so it turned out to be. She explained briefly that she had always wondered what had happened to me and that eventually she had dealt with her anxiety by having me traced through an agency. The implication was that this had happened a little while ago and initially she had been relieved to know that I was still alive and seemingly surviving well enough. More recently, prompted by television programmes she had seen on the implications of genetic inheritance, she had thought I might have anxieties about my origins, which she would be justified in trying to assuage. Hence the family tree and some further details in the letter about my natural father who she had also contacted after many years silence. They both sounded fit, well and likely to live to a ripe old age.

This most recent and authentic version of the truth had the great merit of adding substantial flesh to earlier accounts. When my adoptive mother had died two years earlier I had seen the correspondence with the adoption agency, which had filled out the picture a little. Principally, however, it was instructive for the attitudes it revealed to adoption in the immediate post-war period. On half-size paper, the secretary to the National Adoption Society provided brief details of the child in terms of its birth weight and the simplest antecedents of the natural parents. Thus, I was described as a nice baby, coming recommended by a committee member acquainted with the mother's family, respectable Scottish farming stock. Father, on whom a satisfactory blood test was held, was said to be a 'lawyer', but marriage had not been thought advisable. The prospective parents were instructed to bring a shawl and a basket to the Society's office to take me home for the usual trial period to see if they liked the look of me. Fortunately they had, having been disappointed in an earlier 'offer' who had never been brought to the Office.

This newest version confirmed that my mother was called Smith – a fact that I had often wondered about even though it was her name on the original birth certificate. There was confirmation, too, for another part of the story that I had only heard about when I was 21. My birth mother had turned up at the county court adoption proceedings. As originally told to me by a relative, it had sounded as if consent to the adoption might have been problematic. On the one occasion I had mentioned the incident to my adoptive mother, she had not found it easy to discuss. It seemed certain, therefore, that my natural mother had found it hard to relinquish me and had cared greatly about me. But this new information brought its further frustrations. It had been carefully constructed so there was no immediate way I could contact the sender.

Annoyance was probably the predominant emotion with which I was left at the end of that day. Amazement and curiosity had preceded it. Now, however, I had to face a definite dilemma. Should I try and trace my birth mother? Wasn't the package an invitation to do so despite the careful – too careful – absence of immediately traceable detail? Why had the information come now? Did it mean that there was not much time left, or had she waited until she guessed her appearance would make little difference to my relationship with my adoptive parents? These questions seemed to require that I came off the fence and pursue positively an adventure I had dithered about for a long time.

Our hunt began with the envelope. Although badly smudged, with the aid of our daughter's magnifying glass, we were able to distinguish in the postmark 'Gloucestershire'. It was also apparent from the family tree that my mother, Ethel, had married a Fredrick. This seemed like a combination of names that might not be that hard to find in a voter's register. I had no appreciation of what a daunting task it is to look through the lists for one constituency, never mind the several that the county was likely to contain. So it was to the Family Record Office that our son and I proceeded on a couple of occasions before realising progress on this front was destined to be extremely slow and even then we might easily miss the vital entry. Some of my general concern that I had made the right choice I discussed with the Post Adoption Society of whose existence I had learnt through an article in the *Guardian*. They felt I should look if I wanted to. But ambivalence remained to the extent that it was a year before I finally decided that more definite steps would be needed and I resorted to a tracing agency myself. Within 24 hours and at minimal cost, I had the address and telephone number for which I was looking.

But why the ambivalence? Of course, I had from time to time wondered who my natural parents might be. The question was strongest when I was much younger and could elicit an interesting range of responses if I dropped the fact that I was adopted into conversation. But fairly quickly I had come to the view that whoever my natural parents had been, my adoptive parents obviously thought more of me. They, it should be said, never encouraged such a view, always emphasising that my natural parents had wanted the best for me and, in the circumstances, had operated in the most unselfish manner possible. What those circumstances might have been was, of course, unclear. The end of the war and the possible embarrassment of an unexpected child seemed the most logical conclusion – as it turned out to be but not quite in the manner expected. Over the years curiosity had dwindled and I had no special desire to know more. The discovery that my father was 'a lawyer' briefly rekindled interest but not sufficiently to make any purposive move, until the package arrived. Now added to a revived curiosity was the feeling that I should provide some reassurance that in putting me up for adoption Ethel had made a good decision. I wrote, at last, just before Christmas.

It was obviously the right thing to have done. Letters were quickly exchanged and we arranged to meet. Ethel would come to London and we would meet on Paddington Station. There were no complications and we spent the best part of a day in the excellent café above the concourse exchanging information. Subsequently, we have met Ethel's family – she married in her fifties, but had no other children.

And so to the conundrums: Ethel was mystified as to how I had come to believe my father was a lawyer. He had been an apprentice meal miller. This occupation, I learnt, is seasonal and enquiries in the winter would have found him being described as a sawyer. Ethel felt sure that those from the metropolis would have had little appreciation of rural life and had plumped for the likeliest sounding occupation! As to her appearance at the adoption proceedings, this had indeed occurred. She came to make sure that she liked the look of my new parents. They had met briefly. My mother had suggested that Ethel come for a cup of tea but she had declined, satisfied that I was in safe hands. So why had she had me adopted at all? It was clear that illegitimacy was not the issue. She could easily have married my natural father and had strong feelings for him. Her own family were close and supportive and had survived far worse disasters than an unexpected pregnancy. No – the desire was to escape the harsh tedium of farm life for a career of her own. She had tried to escape at the beginning of the war by volunteering for the armed forces, only to be told she was in a reserved occupation. Now, as the end of the war was in sight, so was the prospect of leaving the land. A baby at this point would have condemned her to further rural confinement. Courageously, Ethel decided to up and go.

Our curiosities were satisfied and possibly a final truth about my adoption established. Ethel's forbearance still seems remarkable, but I feel sure that all my parents would have felt pleased with the outcome, now there are fewer mysteries and anxieties to be borne.

11

LETTER TO A
SOCIAL WORKER

Reflections on mothering

Anonymous

Identity is a complex, ever-changing and multi-dimensional concept in which we are always becoming who we are. The most significant experiences in shaping who I am now are those to do with being a mother, although these are indivisible from my own experiences of having been mothered and indeed, my experiences of being a sister, a friend, a partner, a worker or the many other roles that give my life meaning. I came to mothering through adoption and it is as a black adoptive mother that I write. I do not write for all black mothers although I believe that what I have to say will resonate with many of them, and also with black fathers too. Also, I am sure that there are white people, including mothers and fathers, both those with and without black children, and social workers who share the ideas expressed here. Indeed, I have met many who do and on the occasions where it has happened, have been inspired by their willingness to swim 'against the tide'.

I do not write to you hastily. The ideas presented here are the product of many years of experience and struggle and although much of what I say has to do with social inequality, neither do I write to you in anger. I have dispensed with anger for now, though in the past it has been a useful motivation for action. I write to you because it is important that black women's voices are heard and frankly, it is none too easy to get anyone's attention. Many black women have wearied with trying and instead have directed their efforts towards themselves, each other, their families and communities. There is much to be said for this. It is a survival strategy by which I too have been sustained. It is the fertile ground that is the source of my own growth and it has provided the energy and insights for shared achievements. But, in the spirit of Audre Lorde (Lorde, 1979), I speak to you in the hope that you will open yourself to hearing, for there is much to be put right. Finally, while I do not claim to speak for others, my thoughts have been informed by the many black children and young people, men and women, who share my world.

What I am as an adoptive parent, despite your determined efforts at assessment, has little to do with how you may see me. Assessment, quite apart from other claims made about it, is the process in which your authority carries, promotes and perpetuates dominant discourses on what it means to be a good parent, what kind of family is the right kind of family and how this family should be understood in order that you might match them with a child. It is of concern to me, though of little surprise, that the right kind of family and the good parent are precisely the kinds of people the State wants adoptive families to be. While you have made attempts to be more flexible and creative in your view of families and increasingly, you have been willing to include gay and lesbian, disabled and single parents in your conceptualizations of the 'good' parent, it turns out at the end of the day that you were merely toying with a more inclusive approach. This was, I think, no more that a deviation from the 'norm' – delineating ever more clearly what the normative must be so that when policy makers and politicians demanded a return to the 'old order' it was your compliance rather than resistance that was assured.

The inclusive approach, then, was not a new model at all; it was simply the old model masquerading in contemporary clothes. Don't take this criticism too harshly, adoptive parents are as much a part of this process as you, it benefits many that it should be so. We are often your closest allies; some of us have been you, making these judgements about other adopters. Generally there is little that separates adoptive parents from social workers' views about the right kind of family – the batting is roughly in the same direction. As an adoptive mother I know quite well the games to be played when being assessed – not that there is any deceit in how I portray myself. I simply know that acceptance depends upon the 'fit' between representations and expectations. This may not even be a particularly conscious process for if I am sure of anything, it is that mine is the right kind of family – whatever that is. If it turns out that my projections are as you wish to see me and that this works well for my approval as an adoptive parent, then we are both satisfied. But it is not coincidence that the views of adoptive parents and your assessments marry up in this way, and neither is it due to the gifted insights of the social worker. We all influence and are influenced by those ideas about the good and the bad family, what is best for children and so on.

So, the first thing to make clear is that as an adoptive mother, I am not passive within the assessment process. Also, adoptive parents and social workers are generally not on opposing sides. However, the collusion of adoptive parents with the systems of adoption are not grounds for things remaining as they are and the alliances that are built to protect particular interests cannot mask the ways in which your expressions of power and powerlessness feed into and sustain ideologies which disregard so many.

Social work power, stretching far beyond the bounds of assessment, is a complex matter. It is a mystery to me, for instance, that you abandon all

claims to power in some circumstances and yet wield it with moral right-
eousness in others. Sadly, you often give it up when it matters most that you
use it. This is the case for example, when quite legitimately you question
the racial and cultural appropriateness of approving a white family for the
placement of a black child, but retreat when the going gets tough. The going
is tough on this issue. Politicians of all 'shades'; the 'love is all you need
brigade'; the general public and media, the latter not known for their positive or informed support of black families, make up the motley crew of
bedfellows who raise their collective voices to assert that you, the social
worker, have gone too far. Your decisions about who should and or should
not adopt must be within the government's agenda. That you might, of course,
consider questions of race in the placement of a white child is something you
keep quiet about. Far from this being an irrelevant factor in the placement
of white children, the silence in which you take refuge, simply masks the
fact that such is the depth and extent of consensus in assuming 'white' as
normative that it does not even need to be stated. The assured, taken-for-
granted status of 'whiteness' and its associated assumptions informs assessment, approval and matching processes so pervasively and completely it is
their lifeblood, what then, can there possibly be to question?

This is a reminder to me that positions which benefit the dominant in
society, unlike those of us struggling for recognition in the margins, rarely
need to be defended and would never be subject to charges of ideological
radicalism. It also pointedly serves to underscore, should I be in any doubt,
that my value to British society as a black mother and my contribution to the
lives of black children is considered negligible at worst and minimal at best.

Instead of simply accepting transracial placements as a solution to the
placement needs of black children, perhaps you should question why so much
political and personal energy is invested in supporting this position? Why it
is that opposition is couched as extremism – what deeply held perceptions
of me as a black woman could possibly demand or expect my acquiescence?
Perhaps you should think about the ways in which public research into the
private lives of black transracially placed children subverts the way children
construct and reflect upon their childhood when they grow older. Why it is
that there are no similar public studies of the strengths of black family life
and the ways in which these can provide the protective, nourishing and
empowering factors to achieve the outcomes you have subscribed to for
children (Department of Health, 1999)? Why is it that you want to play down
difference when discussing these issues yet you are among those who have
benefited from the negative representations of difference in wider society just
as surely as black children have not? Why is it that there are so many black
children of mixed (white and black) parentage in local authority care?
What is it that the liberal among you are really saying when you assert that
the 'mixed' family provides the answer? Can you conceive of the possibility
that from where I am sitting, liberalism, despite benevolent intentions, may

not look benign at all but may mask or perpetuate inequalities? And why must the lid be kept on racism, for this is what lies at the root of this discussion? I would like to see it raised up, so I can stamp on its head, and you, can it be that you are prepared to settle for avoiding guilt and discomfort rather than fighting for human rights and social equality?

My comments are not about racial purity. I am not an advocate of clumsy experiments in colour or ethnicity matching and I am not the hostile voice of anti-white rebellion. It is simply that being denuded of the experience of growing and living among black people is an impoverishing experience for black children and for the black people who have so much to give and to gain by becoming their parents. It adds the loss of racial and cultural context to the losses an adopted child may already be dealing with (I make this point in the belief that the experiences of all people must not be reduced to definitive, static or homogenizing notions of race and culture and I also acknowledge that for many black people, culture includes perceptions and experiences as English, Irish, etc.). It reduces black children's opportunities for positive affirmation of themselves as black people and for many black children (this is the case regardless of the 'success' stories you would remind me of) is often the source of internalized racism. For black adults transracially placed as children, it may be the cause of distress and searching in later years.

Perhaps when you have considered all of these questions, you will think about the burden for black children of these weighty matters and also reflect on the messages you give to black adults, for this may help to explain why it is that they do not (in sufficient numbers at any rate) offer themselves as parents to black children in your care?

The power that you have and the ways in which you do or do not exercise it, must surely give you cause for serious reflection? It is not simply that you have power or that I, as a black adoptive mother, do not. Clearly we possess and exercise different levels and different kinds of power at different times. At some stages I have experienced powerlessness, but at the point at which you are unequivocally and finally supporting the adoption of my child, usually the court proceedings, a point long past assessment, approval, matching, 'honeymooning' and so on, I am unlikely to fail and this knowledge alone prevents my feeling powerless. Not so though the other mother in the 'adoption triangle', the birth mother (I cannot remember at what point I switched places with the birth mother and she became the 'other mother' – for many years, this was my position and the change, when it happened, is nothing I could have decreed or preempted). If any group is consistently and systematically disempowered through the processes that take place in order to secure children's future through adoption, then it is the birth parents. The symbol of the triangle to refer to the three parties involved in adoption: the child, the adoptive parents and the birth parents (which in many cases means a single mother), seems very inappropriate given this situation. Implicit in its unspoken 'equilateralism' is the notion that we are all equal stakeholders. However, if the stakes are high for the adoptive parents, then for the birth parents, proceedings which legally, irreversibly and often compulsorily sever their connections with their child, the stakes could not be higher. The relationship between the powerlessness of the birth parent and the power of the social worker is illustrated here:

> She felt discredited as a parent in court because it was proved that she was unworthy. She was too distressed to go back into court after being publicly humiliated. She was shocked that the social services department had presented certain facts as evidence ... [she] felt 'raped' by the exposure of private family affairs – the microscopic attention to detail without putting it in the context of events in their life ... evidence about inadequate provision of food caused great distress ... she had fed her children at her father's house because of her partner's violence. It was therefore true that there was no food in the house but for her the implication that she did not feed her children was very wounding
>
> (Charlton *et al.*, 1998)

The 'unworthiness' of the birth mother is of course heightened by the 'worthiness' of the adoptive mother and very often the evidence of the one is juxtaposed quite literally, against the evidence of the other. I was ecstatic at the adoption of my child; the joy on my face perpetually pours out from the photographs – like liquid sunshine (a little sickly I often think). The tremendous battles we had shared over the years as we struggled to deal with past pains and future fears, were equated in my mind with a protracted, often excruciating labour and the joy in my face is simply the joy of delivery. Of course my child was my child long before the adoption hearing, yet formal affirmation of this was important to us both. I wonder though how we might have managed had it involved a public demonstration of the unworthiness of the woman who had loved him first, loved him still and would remain so important in his life?

As I have stated, my 'worthiness' (or otherwise) as an adoptive parent is tested out through the process of assessment. Yet, I cannot help but feel you are missing the point. The skills you use in order to exercise your powers of disapproval and approval would be of more benefit if they were used to support our reflection on our experiences of mothering and the ways in which we deal with our own childhood losses and pain. This might help us to pause before visiting our ghosts upon our children and it could offer some insights into the strengths and resources we may draw upon to attend to our children's needs.

It was not that I was destined to become a mother by adoption but for some inexplicable reason, it simply occurred to me as the most obvious way to have a child, as 'natural' to me as giving birth biologically. Equally inexplicable is the fact that this was a view never discussed, but understood, unquestioned and accepted by all of my family. It is not that I was unable to conceive this was irrelevant to me – my child would be born to someone else and neither I nor anyone around me ever expected anything different. I retain at the back of my mind some half-baked rationale in the fact that I was named after an aunt who died in childbirth. I repeat it now, as if there is credence in the idea of a spiritual connection with this African woman that provided me with the capacity to love as completely my own, another woman's child, just as someone I hope has loved her child who is of course, my cousin. This all came to me when the adoption agency I first approached asked me my reasons for wanting to adopt. I was stumped, I didn't have any, I just did. Since then I have come to believe that it was my mother, who was not African at all and was in fact a white English woman, whose notion of family and whose capacity to love those who became a part of it has helped to define my own version of mothering. Although born at a time and within a society whose conventions on family life and who could or could not be part of it were rigidly prescribed and upheld, my mother jettisoned herself into the position of being family-less by virtue of her marriage to my father, a black African man. Her own mother, the main source of love in her life, had died when she was a child and so there was no one to prevent this rejection. The resultant exclusion, permanent and total, was an early childhood lesson to me about the negative consequences of being black in Britain. Later, living in Africa and undaunted by previous losses, my mother established a place for herself and for her children within a network of African friends and selected members of my father's family. The 'family' she created was unbounded and unfettered by biological constraints, yet the mutual care-giving and support was so deeply shared that the kinship it engendered sustained my mother until her death. I have never been able to view family through the lens of orthodoxy. Our family has been both fluid and flexible and yet for all that, has maintained a deep feeling of connectedness.

As a black woman, I have often found myself mothered by other black women – English, African, Caribbean and Asian too. They have nurtured me and they have loved me, of this I am absolutely sure. This has helped me in dealing with my own childhood abuses and pains. They have shown me versions of black mothers that are not represented in mainstream society; black mothers with resilience, resourcefulness and humour; black mothers with the determination for making sure that they get the best for black children; and black mothers who have shared in the mothering of my own child and expected that I would do the same for theirs. Their willingness to mother my child meant that the lessons he learned, the boundaries he lived within and the values he came to own were created and sustained in ways that stretched beyond me. This found its most profound expression in his emerging sense of himself as a black child and as he came to know first them and then the black men who were a part of their lives – their sons, fathers, brothers, friends, partners – he was able to imagine the kind of black man he might become. Freed from the limiting and negative representations of black people that were his early experience, his imagination has become boundless and creative. Should you doubt the benefits of self-pride and positive black image to a black child, achieved in the context of loving black adults, it is this that is the basis of health and emotional happiness. As for other achievements, these require not only self-esteem, but also attention to the structural inequalities that thwart our children's potential and ambitions – your social services objectives for children are meaningless without regard to these matters.

I do not suggest that there is some essential or mythical mothering quality that black women have (black people have no need of further stereotypes, even positive ones), I simply share my experiences. Neither do I negate the importance of the contribution of men, both black and white, to the lives of black children. Black fathering in particular is so significant and so under-acknowledged that it requires a chapter of its own and my life has been immeasurably enriched by many of the black fathers I have met, including my own brothers. My focus on black mothering simply represents one particular aspect of parenting.

And so it is that I am left wondering why your assessments seem to miss so much that is rich about what black women have to offer. As for myself, I found in being a mother, and in my attachment to my own mother, awareness of the fundamental importance to my child of rediscovering the past. From somewhere came the resources to face with him and defeat, those early monsters that were truly terrifying – sometimes they lurked in the shadows but at others they jumped on our backs. I knew that my child had his own view of mothering and that his acceptance of me was inextricably linked to those first experiences of being mothered. The wisdom to search came when it was needed, the strength to put aside my own insecurities and to facilitate contact was harder to find, but I held on to a deep-down belief, strengthened by knowing that mothering could be shared and was not possession, that the attachment my child and I had to one another would be strengthened not lessened by this. For some years we lived our lives with more than one mother, and then there came a time when the only mother my child wanted and needed was me. There is no victory or self-satisfaction in this, it is in the way of searching that one often comes to an end, or if not to the end, at least to a point at which one feels ready to stop.

I want you to know that all of this and much more about who I am is knowable, although it is constantly changing. Your assessment simply fixes me in a place where I cannot stay.

References

Charlton, L., Crank, M., Kansara, K. and Oliver, C. (1998), *Still screaming: birth parents compulsorily separated from their children*, Manchester, After Adoption.

Department of Health (1999), *Social services objectives for children*, London, The Stationery Office.

Lorde, A. (1979), An open letter to Mary Daly, in C. Moraga and G. Anzaldua (eds) (1983), *This bridge called my back: writings by radical women of colour*, New York, Kitchen Table: Women of Color Press.

12

ADOPTION AND FAMILY SUPPORT

Two means in pursuit of the same end

Jane Tunstill

Few issues cast such a powerful searchlight across the landscape of child care policy, as the rationale and function of family support. It is a debate capable, where it is permitted, of penetrating even unlikely areas of policy and practice, and of illuminating our understanding of the lengthy child care continuum. And nowhere is this more obviously the case than in the boundary between family support and adoption. It is to the credit of the editors of this volume that a discussion of family support has been allowed across it.

'Family support' is perhaps one of the most contested terms in childcare. By contrast with the concept of adoption, with its apparently precise legal connotations, family support is capable of meaning all things to all people, and its very breadth has probably militated against it being taken as seriously as it should. Even those who drafted the Children Act, 1989, with its emphasis on the need to provide services for children in need, fell short of providing an unambiguous definition of family support, preferring instead to focus on the definition of, and response to, need. Given that need is arguably the most elusive concept within the welfare lexicon, it is no surprise that the political, policy and practice interpretations of family support vary as much as they do. Indeed, as author after author has stressed, family support has to be seen in a wider social policy context, if its scope and limitations are to be fully understood (Hardiker *et al.*, 1996; Holman, 1988; Fox Harding, 1996; Tunstill, 2000). In essence, these social policy questions are those which 'interrogate the "relationship between the needs" generated in civil society and the "services" provided by the state; about what is driving the relationship as a particular "process" and about whether the resulting "outcomes" for children and families are desirable, or even those intended' (Pinkerton, 2000).

However, in spite of all this confusion and complexity, a range of working definitions have been proposed, of which the following are examples:

99

- Any activity or facility provided either by statutory agencies or by community groups or individuals aimed at providing advice and support to parents to help them in bringing up their children (Audit Commission, 1994).
- (It) is about the creation and enhancement, with and for families in need, of locally based (or accessible) activities, facilities and networks, the use of which have outcomes such as alleviated stress, increased self-esteem, promoted parental/carer/family competence and behaviour and increased parental/carer capacity to nurture and protect children (Hearn, 1995, p. 6).
- Family support seeks to promote the child's safety and development and prevent the child leaving the family by reducing stressors in the child and family's life, promoting competence in the child, connecting the child and family members to relevant supports and resources and promoting morale and competence in the parents (Gilligan, 2000, p. 14).

It should also be noted that, in the last few years, a new factor has appeared on the scene in the shape of an emphasis on the concepts of 'parenting' and 'parenting services' (Henricson et al., 2001, p. 18). Approaching family support from this particular angle, with an emphasis on 'parenting deficit', carries certain hazards for the undertaking of family support and preventive work. It could be thought to increase the chances of 'sanctions' rather than 'support' being applied to those who don't make the grade. The response to those parents who fail to do so, may, as opposed to the provision of a broader package of support services of course, include the removal of the child from her/his family; and ultimately of course (in a now, supposedly, shorter time-scale), placement for adoption.

It can be seen from the above quotations that, while approaches to defining family support vary, they almost all point to two essential elements: those services provided on an essentially universal basis, such as health, education and some forms of income support; and those provided on a selective basis, like case-work, home visiting by volunteers, parent education and training, and some forms of day care. The likely reality, as research consistently demonstrates, is that some families need both (Utting, 1995; Buchanan, 1999; Tunstill and Aldgate, 2000), but complications arise with the question of when, how, for how long, to whom; and on the basis of which conditions, these services should be delivered.

Whilst policy at the beginning of the last decade addressed the need to 'refocus' services away from an exclusive concentration on child protection, towards a continuum of child welfare services (Aldgate and Tunstill, 1995; Thoburn et al., 2000), recent government policy has chosen a different emphasis and begun to strike a different balance.

The idea of a continuum between *children in need* and *children in need of protection* has been replaced by a greater and very welcome emphasis on universal services, through which the reduction of social exclusion is largely to be pursued. There may be hybrid versions of this, such as Sure Start, which is universal within a selective or targeted high need area. However, for a minority of families this new world may carry problematic implications. It is far from clear what should/will happen if and when those universal approaches appear to prove, at least in the short term, inadequate. Put bluntly, are the most 'needy' families – emotionally and socially as well as materially – now at risk of falling through the gap between *universal family support* on the one hand, and, if it fails to work, the draconian step of *having their children permanently removed* on the other? There are some grounds for such pessimism in recent policy statements on adoption, including, for example, the new national Adoption Standards (Department of Health, 2001a).

'Every child wants to grow up in a stable and loving family. The need to strengthen support for the family has been recognised in a range of government policies designed to promote healthy living and to combat poverty and social exclusion, particularly amongst children. Where children cannot live with their birth parents, the important but difficult task of finding them a new family falls to local councils and voluntary adoption agencies. Adoption is the means of giving children an opportunity to start again in a legally permanent family' (Foreword to the Adoption Standards by Jacqui Smith, Minister for Health).

These adoption standards are certainly underpinned by a clear and explicit set of values; including the importance of supporting the family.

- Children are entitled to grow up as part of a loving family which can meet their needs during childhood and beyond.
- It is best for children where possible to be brought up by their own birth family.

However, the exact nature of the standards themselves departs sharply from the tone set in these opening sections. Standards one and two, which might reasonably given the earlier statements, have required local authorities to provide evidence of a concerted effort to enable the child to 'be brought up by their own birth family' skip that stage altogether. Instead, they read as follows:

- Children whose birth family cannot provide for them with a secure, stable and permanent home are entitled to have adoption considered for them.
- Whenever plans for permanence are being considered, they will be made on the basis of the needs of each looked after child, and within the following time-scales . . .

So, in reality therefore, there is no procedural mechanism, such as a 'Set of Standards for Family Support', to put into practice the stated emphasis on the importance of the birth family, nor even a single standard within the Adoption Framework, to ensure that every possible effort has been made to enable the child to grow up in her/his birth family. If adoption and family support really are to be seen as allies in a battle for the best interests of the child, then this is not a promising beginning.

Why might these omissions be important? Why should there be an equivalent strategic plan for family support with the same legal clout as Adoption Standards? Why is the sustained and widespread availability of family support as central to the welfare of children as the opportunity to be adopted? Perhaps the most import question is 'can well-resourced and highly regarded family support provision co-exist alongside a robust policy aimed at increasing the role of adoption?'

The following section indicates the general line of argument in response. It is based on the assumption that the legal and administrative shape of children's services should genuinely reflect each of the three principles below. All three have been acknowledged as essential within current statutory initiatives and are cited by those who support an increased rate of adoptions. All three point unequivocally to the need for family support to be accorded a central place in child care policy, as well as to the dangers of replacing it with ill-thought out and hasty attempts to increase the rate of adoption.

The starting point for arguing the centrality of family support has to be the requirement for child welfare policy and practice to be, first and foremost, child centred.

'Fundamental to establishing whether a child is in need and how those needs should be met is that the approach must be child centred' (Framework for the Assessment of Children in Need and their Families, Department of Health, 2000). Indeed this reiterates the requirement of Section 17 in Part 111 of the Children Act, 1989, to safeguard and promote the welfare of children in need by providing a range and level of services. It is impossible to adopt a child centred approach without taking account of the family environment into which the child is born, and having done so, family support can and should be delivered in a child centred way. Practitioners and policy makers often overlook the very high level of flexibility, in terms of both content and time-scale, inherent in family support. There is nothing automatically child centred about foreshortening the provision of support to a family, in the interests of meeting bureaucratic guidelines, and increasing ratings such as those in Quality Protects (Department of Health, 1998).

Almost as important as the requirement for child centred services is the second conviction that such services must be rooted in an understanding of child development (Department of Health, 2000). There is a consensus in the research literature (Department of Health, 2001b) that children have a range of developmental needs; and that these may change over time. These needs will include those they have in common, such as for food, shelter, social interaction, health care and intellectual stimulation ; but also those special needs, manifested by a minority, such as children with physical or learning disabilities or emotional or behavioural problems.

The frustration of these developmental needs, especially in combination, is closely associated with seriously impaired life chances (Rutter, 1984; Rutter and Madge, 1976). However, research also points to the fact that, given the right opportunities, many children can overcome early disadvantage (Pilling, 1990). Family support has a highly developed compensatory capacity, exemplified by services such as high quality early years provision and a recent range of pre-delinquency programmes (DfES, 1999; Utting *et al.*, 1993). It also has a powerful 'protective' capacity and can, as research consistently demonstrates, reduce a range of risks to children within their birth families. It can 'serve as one important strand in the range of strategies necessary to counteract the toxic effects on personal, family and neighbourhood life of social exclusion' (Gilligan, p. 15).

The third argument is in many ways a political as well as a professional or theoretical one. Ecological theory has a central place within current government policies on the assessment of children (Department of Health, 2000). The symmetry between family support and an ecological way of working has already been flagged up in the two points above. Ecological theory argues that we can only understand individuals in the context of the environment in which they live, that is to say in terms of the social and material resources to which they have access, at the levels of family, friends, neighbourhood and society (Jack, 2001). Issues such as poverty; housing; health inequalities and social integration are all subsumed within this framework. Ecological theory has very clear political implications, and in particular, complements the current government's stress on addressing social exclusion, of which current child welfare policies are an important aspect. Ensuring the provision of a range of family support resources is one obvious way in which to achieve social inclusion. In tandem with universal services, such as health and education, which may meet the needs of a majority of children, it can ensure that more complex and/or individual circumstances are addressed in order to achieve optimum outcomes for children.

The brief discussion above, has attempted to draw attention to the indispensable role which family support plays in the lives of children in need. Its capacity to facilitate positive outcomes for children has been consistently demonstrated by research. It also complements the social policy value base of the current government. However, there are currently worrying indications that the strategy of adoption is being presented as a premature answer to complex child and family situations. There is some suggestion, borne out by current political statements about adoption, that some children will find themselves caught up in the adoption process, sooner rather than later, instead of them and their birth families being offered access to specialised, as well as universal, family support resources. It ought, on the basis of the theories referred to above, to be possible for adoption and family support to survive and indeed thrive within the same child care continuum. This will only be the case if strenuous effort is made to avoid the apparently easy option of premature adoptions. Both adoption and family support interventions need careful planning, implementation, adequate resourcing and rigorous evaluation. Easy options, after all, usually only exist in the eye of the beholder.

References

Aldgate, J. and Tunstill, J. (1995), *Making sense of section 17: implementing services for children in need within the Children Act, 1989*, London, HMSO.

Audit Commission (1994), *Seen but not heard: co-ordinating community health and social services for children in need*, London, HMSO.

Buchanan, A. (1999), *What works for troubled children? Family support for children with emotional and behavioural problems*, Barkingside, Barnardos.

Department of Health (1998), *Quality protects circular: transforming children's services*, London, Local Authority Circular (LAC(98)29).

Department of Health (2000), *Framework for the assessment of children in need and their families*, London, Department of Health.

Department of Health (2001a), *The Children Act now: messages from research*, London, The Stationery Office,

Department of Health (2001b), *National adoption standards for England*, London, DOH.

Department for Education and Skills (1999), *Sure Start: making a difference for children and families*, Sudbury, DfES.

Fox Harding, L. (1996), *Family, state and social policy*, Basingstoke, Macmillan.

Gilligan, R. (2000), Family support: issues and prospects in J. Canavan, P. Dolan, and J. Pinkerton, (eds) *Family support: direction from diversity*, London, Jessica Kingsley Publishers.

Hardiker, P., Exton, K. and Barker, M. (1996), *A framework for analysing services, Childhood Matters*, vol. 2, Background Papers, London, HMSO.

Hearn, B. (1995), *Child and family support and protection: a practical approach*, London, National Children's Bareau.

Henricson, C., Katz, I., Mesie, J., Sandison, M. and Tunstill, J. (2001), *National mapping of family services in England and Wales: a consultation document*, London, National Family and Parenting Institute.

Holman, B. (1988), *Putting families first: prevention and child care*, Basingstoke, Macmillan.

Jack, G. (2001), Ecological perspectives in assessing children and families, in Horwath, J. (eds) *The child's world: assessing children in need*, London, Jessica Kingsley Publishers.

Pilling, D. (1990), *Escape from disadvantage*, Brighton, The Falmer Press.

Pinkerton, J. (2000), Emerging agendas for family support in J. Canavan, P. Dolan, and J. Pinkerton (eds) *Family support: direction from diversity*, London, Jessica Kingsley Publishers.

Rutter, M. (1984), Continuities and discontinuities in socioemotional development: empirical and conceptual perspectives, in R. N. Emde and R. J. Harman (eds) *Continuities and discontinuities in development*, New York, Plenum.

Rutter, M. and Madge, N. (1976), *Cycles of disadvantage*, London, Heinemann.

Thoburn, J., Wilding, J. and Watson, J. (2000), *Family support in cases of emotional neglect*, London, The Stationery Office.

Tunstill, J. (2000), Child care, in M. Hill (ed.), *Local authority social services: an introduction*, Oxford, Blackwell.

Tunstill, J. and Aldgate, J. (2000), *Services for children in need: from policy to practice*, London, Stationery Office.

Utting, D. (1995), *Family and parenthood: supporting families, preventing breakdown*, York, Joseph Rowntree Foundation.

Utting, D., Bright, J. and Henricson, C. (1993), *Crime and the family; improving child rearing and preventing delinquency*, London, Family Policy Studies Centre.

Part III

LIFE AFTER ADOPTION

INTRODUCTION

The making of an Adoption Order by a Court used to be regarded as the final stage of the adoption process. While it remains a defining moment, it is now viewed as only one milestone in the development of a child in care who had needs before adoption, and who will have equally strong needs afterwards, possibly for the rest of its childhood and potentially through into adulthood. Adoption agencies are therefore required to stay involved and to support the adoption in different ways, for example by helping to formulate an education plan for the child (school matters!) and to ensure the resources are in place for it to be delivered, to arrange respite care, or therapeutic support (Lowe *et al.*, 1999). It is a mistake to think that post-adoption services are merely about arranging contact or information exchanges between a child and its birth parents, or just staying in touch for the first year 'until things settle down', and then having a clean break. Life in many adoptions today is just not like that.

Post-adoption services are now as important as pre-adoption assessments and matching processes, but they are still non-existent in many parts of the UK, despite being a statutory responsibility.

> The lack of developed and comprehensive post-adoption services emerge universally. Though many councils have plans to develop services or have already appointed development workers or post-adoption support workers, there is little in place to ensure the necessary support and assistance to adoptive families in the long term. For a significant number, the lack of a post-adoption service is the main reason for delaying the final stage in the adoption process – the seeking of an adoption order.
>
> (Department of Health, 2000)

'Love is not enough' when caring for troubled children – skills in behaviour management, to name but one, are vital (BBC, 2000). Equally, long-term non-involvement after placement by an adoption agency is not enough.

A good post-adoption service will:

- Ensure adopters are aware of how to access their local post-adoption service, for example by providing an information pack to all adopted children and adults.
- Ensure the adoption has been kicked off properly, with due consideration having been given to whether an adoption allowance was needed, whether a housing adaptation was needed if the adopted child has a profound disability, and whether the adopters have clear, comprehensive written information about the child they are looking after.
- Make a local support group available for adopters.
- Use adoption partnership contracts, between the placing agency and the adopter/s, which set out the areas of future placement support, with a built in annual review mechanism.
- Have an adoption link-worker available who knows the child and the family and who is prepared to offer support at the time of crisis, and to link the adoptive family into professional services like the child and adolescent mental health service, and school support services.
- Have an arrangement in place for independent mediation when contact arrangements go wrong or are challenged.
- Review each adoption breakdown at the adoption panel.
- Provide a similarly accessible service for birth relatives, so they can stay in touch, deposit information about changes in their circumstances, etc.

The first major post-adoption service was the Post-Adoption Centre in London, which opened in 1986, although several adoption agencies had been providing services since the 1970s. From the outset, the centre was responding to allcomers.

> Although the work with adoptive families is probably the most time-consuming, and they are the ones we are most likely to take on for a series of sessions, they represented only 21 per cent of the total enquiries or requests for help in the centre's first year of operation. 44 per cent were adopted adults, and 15 per cent were birth parents. The balance were other relatives, most often brothers and sisters, and sometimes grandparents (Hill and Shaw, 1998).

Post-adoption services also have to reach out to birth parents. Contact between a birth parent and their child can be face to face, at intervals varying from weekly, which is highly unusual, to annually; or through letters, cards, presents, audiotapes or videotapes, photographs, e-mails or phone calls. Indirect contact can also be made using an intermediary agency or individual as a postbox. For birth parents, contact mitigates a sense of loss, can ease the pain, especially knowing their child is OK; it can reduce feelings of powerlessness and help the birth parent move on, which is important in terms of the emotional framework a birth parent brings to future parenting; and can increase the acceptance of the adoption, however mixed feelings are.

For adoptive parents, contact can reduce their fear of the birth parents; reduce their fantasy of how attached the child is to their birth parent/s; and can lead to a greater understanding of the child; and can reinforce support for the adoption (Department of Health, 2001). Where trails have gone cold, tracing agencies can often help. Reality can beat fantasy some times. Allison Perkin, adopted by a teacher in Dorset, found out at the age of 32 that her birth father was Bobby King, one of Britain's most famous bank robbers (*Guardian*, 20 December 2000).

Support for birth mothers is a vital part of a comprehensive adoption service, not least because birth mothers who have lost children often go on to have more children. 'What do you say to your four-year-old who went into care because you neglected him or because your partner abused him?', a birth parent asked one of the editors. After Adoption supports women who have had their children removed from them, including a project to support women in Styal Prison in Cheshire. As Maureen Crank, director of After Adoption, said: 'We're seeing a picture of people succeeding when support and parenting training is put in. Some of the mothers were very young and in abusive relationships. They do grow up and mature' (quoted, *Community Care*, 7–13 December 2000). After Adoption advocates the establishment of an independent national support and counselling service for birth parents.

The Post-Adoption Action Group believes that 'any review of current adoption legislation must incorporate a substantive review of Sections 50 and 51 of the Adoption Act, 1976, to ensure compatibility with all Convention Rights. They believe that all adopted persons and their birth relatives should have a statutory right of access to information which makes it possible for them to locate each other. Many campaigners believe that the law discriminates against people adopted before the right to trace was introduced, because they have no rights of access to information unless the adoption agency who handled their case decides they can, or unless they secure a court order requiring an adoption agency to disclose specific information.

A number of landmark cases confirm the trend towards information about adoption becoming open and accessible to all parties. In 2001, Linda Gunn-Russo, the daughter of an American GI and a British woman, won a High Court action which ordered the Nugent Care Society to give her access to all the information they held about her early life. Whilst more local authorities like Westminster City Council are facilitating access to information for birth mothers who relinquished their children a generation ago, many adoptees continue to have problems gaining full access to their original adoption records. In many countries, access is still totally denied, despite human rights conventions and legislation. For many adopted people, seeing their file and finding out exactly what happened to them, and why, is the key to them being able to deal with their past satisfactorily and, if need be, move on.

Contact for some children though has its downside. Contact orders, even in an adoption, are sometimes granted to abusive parents, who continue to threaten children in their new placements, often subtly and covertly. There are some parents whose contact should be terminated permanently, not just because of the abuse they inflicted on a child, but because of their continuing capacity to seriously threaten the child's emotional and psychological welfare in the period leading up to and after contact visits or phone calls. Children's needs vary over time, and they are mostly highly resilient, but in general, there is no evidence that contact decreases stability, and most children want as much or more contact. According to Thomas and Beckford, half of the children who had contact with birth parents were satisfied, half wanted more contact, and only 1 wanted less contact (Thomas and Beckford, 1999). Adoption is no different from second marriages, whereby children want to see their previous parent as much as they can, however badly they have behaved.

Our book features some special adopters, marvellous people, like Deborah Savidge and Hugh Maloney, who have helped children with troubled early lives resume a normal pattern of development. Their stories demonstrate that there are scarcely any children who are unadoptable by nature, if the right adopters can be found and if the placements are properly supported. Gill Gray describes how concurrent planning works. Julia Feast and David Howe discuss the communication strategies needed for more open adoptions. Val Forrest and Pam Hodgkins set out ways in which post-adoption support can be given to all stakeholders in the adoption process. Other contributors, like Veronica Dewan, speak of what happens when poor placements are made, the lifelong repercussions of which can be devastating for the individuals and those close to them. Finally in this section, Jane French writes about marriage to an adoptee who never felt he belonged anywhere. French's story is a reminder that adoptive parents are not innately superior to birth parents, as politicians from all major parties suggested during the 1990s when debating the question of state support for single parents, particularly financial support. Good and loving parenting, by whoever offers it, is what counts.

References

BBC (2000), *Love is not enough*, London, BBC Publications.

Department of Health (2000), *Adopting changes: survey of local authority adoption services*, London, Department of Health.

Hill, M. and Shaw, M. (1998), *Signposts for adoption, policy, practice and research issues*, London, BAAF.

Lowe, N., Murch, M., Borkowski, M., Weaver, A. and Beckford, V., with Thomas, C. (1999), *Supporting adoption: reframing the approach*, London, British Agencies for Adoption and Fostering.
Thomas, C. and Beckford, V. with Lowe, N. and Murch, M. (1999), *Adopted children speaking*, London, British Agencies for Adoption and Fostering.

13

ADOPTION

Perspectives from family members

Deborah Savidge and Hugh Maloney

Deborah

We were in our thirties when we got together, enthusiastic to have our own family. We were both established enough at work to have flats and mortgages and few financial worries. The biological time bomb was beginning to tick and brothers, sisters and friends were reproducing at a rapid rate. It wasn't the only thing on our minds, however. We had bought our first sailing cruiser and were having incredible adventures exploring the coasts of Britain and North Europe. We were also involved in a self-build group aiming to build our own house in central London as well as work and an active social life!

Hugh

Late thirties is a more accurate description of me at the time. Deborah and I met through work. She was running a very successful inner city youth club and was part of the recruitment panel for a youth-crime reduction project I was interested in. I got the job and because our experiences and views were similar we became natural allies. We started to see each other outside work and nature soon took its course. In talking about our future together, having a family was high on our agenda and we did all we could to make it happen. We were determined rather than desperate. Our lives were busy and we kept our options open.

Deborah

Anyway, no pregnancy occurred so we turned to technology – the IVF solution. We thought ourselves really lucky to have this option and were treated with great care in a dimly-lit basement by the dedicated staff at Bart's Hospital. My rabidly Socialist GP lectured me on the cost of the treatment and how this necessarily deprived his other patients and I carried large containers of my urine around at work in some modern equivalent to a knights of the round table task.

After four attempts, we called it a day. I was 40, the house was nearly built and the next boat, a round-the-world cruiser, was at the drawing board stage.

Hugh

Deborah remained characteristically calm and positive throughout the IVF treatment. Fortunately natural caution prevented us from expecting too much. When it failed we continued to plan for a future without children while at the same time investigating the possibility of becoming adoptive parents. We pressed on with building a family house and began preparation for a three-year sailing cruise. The house would be our family home if children arrived or a source of income to fund the cruise if they didn't.

Deborah

It was my Mum and sister dying that decided us on the next course – adoption. Suddenly my family was growing smaller and there seemed to be gaps that needed filling. There also loomed the Big One, the ever-growing spectre of the transience of life. The adoption process had its ups and downs. At various times, we were told that we were too old, too busy, had too many flats (one each), or too many cars (one each) to adopt, but perseverance won through and a four-year-old Sara arrived.

Sara was put up for adoption because of a history of abuse and because social services and the courts were not convinced the abuse would end. The adoption was contested by her birth mother and a Guardian ad Litem was appointed by the court to collect evidence from the parties involved. She caused us a worrying moment by announcing that we had too many books and that our hospitality was considerably less than Sara's birth mother's. While we had merely offered her a cup of tea, Sara's birth mother had supplied 'a whole table full of food'.

Despite this gross oversight on our part, the court did decide in our favour and the adoption went through. Meanwhile, Sara had started school and the celebration of her adoption coincided with her first parents' evening at the local C of E primary where her teacher took us to one side with the dreaded words, 'You will be disappointed to hear', our hearts were in our boots, 'Sara is a leg swinger in Church'.

Sara was delightful (still is) and very anxious to please (less so now). At first, she worryingly acquiesced to any suggestion, so you can imagine our delight after 6 weeks or so when she refused to do something. We danced around celebrating the first but by no means the last, 'No. I won't'. Friends and family all loved her and she took to weekends on the boat like a duck to water. On one memorable occasion, as her parents turned green and sickly in a stormy sea which forced us back into harbour she was happily drawing with pencils and crayons, having cunningly jammed herself into a position where she was not being thrown about.

We adored Sara from the start and felt a 'complete family'. Work moved ahead on the house and our plans for the big cruise continued, when out of the blue, we received a call from our social worker–fairy godmother – 'would Sara like a baby brother?' How could anybody say no? Again we were locked into a protracted legal procedure without a certain outcome.

A year later we moved into our almost completed house and I was about to take early retirement at 42, the redundancy money buying a steel hull for our round-the-world cruise. I finished work on the Friday and we picked up Oliver and Thomas the Tank Engine the following day. He was 18 months old, just walking and as sunny as the day is long unless I vacuumed the house or he was faced with anything that remotely resembled fruit or vegetables. We had struck lucky again and Sara and Oliver soon became inseparable companions,

But why was I feeling so sick and why had my periods stopped? Surely a few disturbed nights couldn't have such devastating physical effects? I dragged myself around to our GP who said I might be pregnant. 'Unlikely' I scoffed, handing over more urine to be tested.

Phoebe was born in October and I joined an elite club of those who had retired before giving birth. Five days later we were before a judge – this time putting the legal seal on Oliver's adoption. Within a couple of years we had acquired three children and a houseful of toys, Disney videos and Lego. The world cruise was put on hold.

Hugh

Adopting the children was a lengthy process involving more cul-de-sacs than journeys completed. It could have easily become a stressful even demeaning experience and it certainly helps to stand back from it all occasionally and look at the funny side. We felt the social work staff were sometimes too young and a little out of their depth. It didn't help them or us that the assessment criteria at the time were too worthy and prone to trendy dogma. However we came across only one case of obvious incompetence and it all turned out OK. In the end we were lucky. We survived unscathed and came out with a family. Others weren't so fortunate.

Like most people on the receiving end of the adoption agencies at that time, we have some pretty firm views about our experiences and about how the selection processes we were put through could have been improved. Since then changes have being made in the regulations, hopefully for the better, but that is another issue. I wanted to write about what happened to us afterwards, about the process of adoptive parenting. I find this much harder to do.

When the two babies arrived everything changed. No amount of fore-warning could have prepared me. Our unfinished house was suddenly full of elderly female relatives and equipment. Adopting a quiet five-year-old was one thing, but the addition of the other two was something else. The babies proved to be unbelievably time consuming. All plans for travel quickly went out the window. I suddenly had family to love and care for and for the first time in my life I had to think seriously about making more than just enough money to support myself. We now had only one salary.

Now, a decade on, when asked about being an adoptive parent and the experience of adoption I tend to forget about the intervening ten years. I think back to the period of endless adoption assessments and of court procedures. What has been happening since then is just family life.

We have been lucky. I would defy anybody to live with and parent our adopted two and not love them. They are terrific. Thinking of other factors which may have helped: both Debbie and I come from sizable, stable and loving families so we know about living together successfully; our own extended families have all taken very naturally to Sara and Oliver so there is depth as well as substance in their family relationships; both of us had worked successfully with children before, particularly teenagers so we are aware of some of the pitfalls; we were fortunate to have followed expert advice and have always been completely open about the adoption; also, Debbie and I just do get on well together. This is how it is for us but I don't doubt that successful adoptive parents can just as easily come from very different backgrounds and experiences.

People often want to know whether or not being father to Sara and Oliver is more problematic than being a father to Phoebe, our natural child? The answer has to be 'no', from what I have seen so far. That said, it is not entirely the same either. There is sometimes something physically familiar or some common characteristic about Phoebe, which I suddenly recognise. This happens with the others as well with say, learned phrases, a certain way of looking, but not as often. Sara, Oliver and Phoebe all have qualities special to themselves and each child has its own set of unique relationships with us. I'm sure our love is just as strong for all three. Of course the normal family problems crop up occasionally, but apart perhaps from the odd event in Sara's earlier years, there have been no significant problems with any of the children that can be attributed directly to adoption. No matter how I look at it, our family life and the relationships we have with our children seem no different to those of other families around us.

Though now small in the overall scheme of things Sara, who was an abused child before coming to us, had some catching up to do particularly in areas such as: self confidence; trust in others; ability to show affection; concen-tration and also in some confusion between acquired and actual memories. Fortunately, twelve years on, little if any of these remain. She enjoys family and school and after excellent GCSEs is currently immersed in her A-levels.

She has some lovely friends and a comfortable low-key social life. She still feels she will not want to trace her birth mother.

Oliver came with far less baggage. He was adopted at a much younger age than Sara and can remember nothing before living with us. He enjoys life at home, is very loyal to the family and often great fun to be with. He has a good social life but is less keen on school work. All three get on well together and Oliver is particularly good with Phoebe, who is the most impetuous. Oliver quite likes the cache of being 'adopted', particularly the thought of having another mother somewhere. He says he is keen to re-establish the relationship when the time comes although he understands she may not be able to do so. How will we feel when he does? I don't know, let's see. We have always known this to be part of the deal and so far it has all worked wonderfully well for us.

Deborah

We have been asked if we feel differently about our own child and of course we do. There is a recognition of certain personality traits. Sometimes we are almost startled by a 'Yes, I know exactly how you feel' empathy, but although it is a different feeling, it is not huge nor does it lessen the emotional ties with Oliver and Sara.

We wanted to make a family and now with three children we have. Our objective was to make sure that they cared for each other and became friends. We have loved them lots, told them off when we had to and really they did the rest for themselves. They bickered and argued and cared and shared, are jealous and proud of each other and have each developed their own personalities. To us they seem very different but a new teacher at their primary school was surprised to learn of their varied backgrounds, 'they all behave in similar ways', she said.

I find it hard to describe family life. It has such a momentum of its own that the last ten years have flown by despite having been full to bursting with achievements, disappointments, activities and fun. The future will bring other challenges as Sara and Oliver meet or do not meet up with their birth families. We hope that they will always be there for each other.

Sara

I am now 16 and have been part of the family for 12 years. To be honest, the first four years of my life are a complete blank and there are not even any photographs of me at this age so all my memories are tied in with my parents and later Oliver and Phoebe. This means that my life really begins at four and that is quite strange, Most of the time I am not really aware of being adopted although I've always known about it and I do have a great friend from Primary School who was also adopted so I can discuss any feelings and matters that arise with her. That sounds a bit serious and actually we do very little talking on the subject. Some instances trigger the fact that I am different like Parents Evenings at School when family likenesses are obvious or other people's perception of adopted children as when, after I talked about adoption in class, the teacher commented how brave I was! So in a way I feel like two different people. I remember Phoebe being born but with Oliver one day he wasn't there but the next day he was.

Because we have different birth parents it had always seemed important that we should not only be brother and sisters but also friends. I do consider myself really lucky. Some people do not get a second chance with parents, I did.

Oliver

Being adopted means that in some way I am different. I tend to only tell a few people I think I can trust about it but sometimes this goes wrong and everybody gets to know. It makes me the centre of attention for a while and I am asked the dumbest questions like 'Do you hate your parents?' They also might say 'You're so unlucky' or 'You're not normal'. I feel OK about everyone in my family. Can I go back to the computer now?

Phoebe

As a 10-year-old girl and younger than my brother or sister I cannot remember as I wasn't alive when my brother and sister were being adopted. However, now when I say my brother and sister are adopted, the answers are a bit like this 'Really? You must really hate them' or 'Oh my God, I feel really sorry for you' I don't feel as if I should hate them though. To me they are just like any other brother or sister. Sometimes I find it weird when people say that I look like my sister.

Maybe, as I am just a child I should not give hints to adults about adoption. However I feel that you should not keep from your child that she or he is adopted as I think that if you give this news later on in life especially in the teenage years it may cause upset and a breakdown in trust. You may have different views. I think adoption is a good choice especially if you don't want to be kept up day and night for one or two years or hate the idea of changing nappies.

I feel much the same as anyone else would towards a brother and sister. I never feel as though they shouldn't have been adopted. My feelings will never change for they grew up with me as my brother and sister and therefore they always will be.

14

A TRUER IMAGE

Veronica Dewan

I wish this narrative recounting my transracial adoption in 1957 was of historical interest only. But, in 2001, I am aware that the experiences of many young transracially placed people are comparable to my own. Adoption into families that deny the existence or impact of racism on their lives can be a noxious combination. Members of my birth and adoptive families have felt defeated by prejudices and ideologies linked to class, religion, nationality and ethnicity. Current adoption policies encourage placement of black and mixed race children with parents who are not committed to confronting and challenging racism, thereby taking serious risks with their mental and physical health. I have survived to tell my story. Others have not.

My birth parents met as students in London travelling on the Circle Line. My father had arrived the previous day from New Delhi, having been awarded a Nehru Scholarship to continue his legal studies. My mother from County Mayo in Ireland had been in London for three years and was on leave prior to retaking her nursing exams. Both looking for adventure, their brief passionate fling in a hotel in Holland Park led to my conception.

His passion led to a solicitor's letter denying paternity. Her passion led to humiliation, a painful separation and denial. She was certain her farming family would reject her if she revealed her secret. She was told by the catholic nuns that adoption was the only solution, they said it was unthinkable for my mother to bring up a mixed race child; it would be a constant reminder of her sin. With no understanding or offer of support, she took me to London and handed me to the Catholic Rescue Society.

My adoptive parents had been married five years and my adoptive mother had major gynaecological difficulties. Lonely and isolated, away from her family in Dublin, my adoptive parents lived in a rural part of southern England. They were poor: he was an agricultural worker, and she could not find work. Upon seeing an advertisement about fostering in *The Universe*, a Catholic newspaper – she thought this would give her the chance of mothering as well as being remunerated. My adoptive father only discovered her plan when he arrived home to find a social worker there. The adoption society subsequently wrote to say I was only available for adoption, not fostering, or

I would be sent to an institution. My adoptive parents travelled to London to collect me. It was 1957 and I was six weeks old.

We all experienced prejudice: my mother, who was a good neighbour, was called racist names such as thick Paddy; my father, a diligent working-class English man, was patronised and exploited. My parents, defeated by the injustice in their own lives, were not able to support me to deal with experiences of racism from teachers in primary school or with class prejudices at the convent grammar school. There was minimal input from social services. The only condition of my adoption was for me to be brought up as Catholic like my birth mother. It was only as an adult that I learned my biological father was a Punjabi Hindu and that my grandmother was a Pathan – ironically, a well known family planning expert. Regrettably, in my childhood, this information about my origins was considered to be of no importance.

At fourteen, I was sent to an approved school for two years. Running away from home, truanting from school, taking drugs, becoming pregnant: the rebellion happened very quickly. It was precipitated by a total breakdown in the relationship with my adoptive mother. From my early memories she was depressed, unable to counteract the anti-Irish racism both in and out of the home. She could not support me. Her untreated depression gradually led to frequent rages, occasional physical violence but mainly emotional threats that she would leave me because I was not her child but 'the child of a whore'. Many times she threatened to take my life and her own. She said she could love other children but not me, that I was responsible for the family poverty and – when I was eight – for her mother's death. My father refused to believe my word against my mother's. The racial abuse I received from neighbours and at school was also denied by my father who told me I was English now and simply making up stories to get attention.

A Welsh teacher told the rest of my class that I cheated to get a high mark for a simple arithmetic test: 'This is what happens with Indians, they are sly and deceitful and not to be trusted'. At seven, deeply humiliated, I considered different ways to kill myself. My first suicide attempt occurred when I was twelve. My mother stormed out of the house because I brought home a tin of curry powder. I was trying to find out who I was and where I belonged – confused and embarrassed that being Irish was also 'bad'.

The Beatles began visiting India. I became a 'hippie'. I took acid, speed, barbiturates, lots of weed and stopped going to school. My sexual activities were 'explained' by the social worker to my parents. 'Indian girls are married with children by this age.' My 'delinquency' developed as psychiatrists, the police and social workers became involved in my life. My pregnancy at thirteen was terminated and my parents handed me back into care. The support we all should have received through my childhood was absent but as the mixed race adoptee I was seen as and believed myself to be the source of the problem.

Released from the approved school at sixteen, I started to deny my Indian and Irish identity. I became the exotic plaything of a man in his forties and moved to France. It was more difficult there for people to place me and I passed sometimes for Mediterranean or South American. But my partner became concerned that I was 'starting to look like an Algerian' and told me to stay out of the sun. I returned to England after three years, with a French accent.

I had married a white English middle-class man and we had been together five years. I was absorbed in and into his middle-class family; they liked my French connection. It seemed like a good defence at the time, and I felt protected by them. I worked in tourism at an airport, welcoming visitors to a Britain that was unwelcoming to me. Following the protests in Brixton in 1981 I started to find my voice in this English family. They were shocked when I expressed disgust at my father-in-law's racist attitudes. My marriage ended quickly in 1982, the protection was gone and I was alone with myself again. I took a massive overdose but survived to move to Paris and organise my first visit to India. I needed a family.

I had contacted the adoption society in 1979 where I learned that my birth mother lived in North America. I was dissuaded from pursuing this information. In 1983 I went to India where I had an address for my biological father but he wasn't there – he was living in London!

When my birth mother arrived from the States in 1985, our respective fantasies were played out briefly while truth simmered beneath the surface. Sent to a Catholic mother and baby home in Grayshott, Surrey, my birth mother had told her brothers she was in hospital having her appendix removed. I was the 'appendix' who was introduced to them nearly thirty years later.

My birth mother was distressed that I had traced my Indian father only weeks before. She was shocked to find me in a relationship with a South Asian man, and distraught that I had not grown into the charming and wealthy English woman of her fantasies. She was not the passionate, artistic and carefree woman of my dreams. I was unprepared for the surges of anger I felt towards her. We struggled hard to retain the relationship.

Eventually I left my partner. I became childlike, unable to look after myself. I wanted to be totally dependent on my mother. She wished I was still the six-week-old baby whom she could mould in her own likeness. But I refused to obey her when my adulthood re-emerged. We were in dangerous territory and much of that time we spent in Los Angeles where racial wounds were raw following the police beating of Rodney King. I last saw my birth mother in Los Angeles the day after the riots broke out.

Perhaps my relationship with my birth mother would have been easier if I had known about my Punjabi Indian heritage earlier in my life, had been given support and access to my cultural background and had been able to depend on people to help me deal with racism. But I had learnt only a short time earlier of my Punjabi heritage and it was that missing piece of me that needed to be filled. My mother's prejudiced views of Indian people, her overt racism towards African Americans and my internalised racism in relation to my Irish identity caused many confrontations between us.

My biological father's fantasy was that I would be a boy. A solicitor with many friends and clients, he was also an alcoholic with a failing practice. He needed someone to trust and I started working for him. I wanted so much to be loved by him but when he said I was the only one who could help him out of the mess he was in, I couldn't bear his dependence on me. It was too distressing after having been abandoned by him. I left after a few months to do a full time law degree. I was starting to crack up. Two years later he died of cancer.

In 1988 I had an abortion. The father of the child was my South Asian partner of five years. He was a lawyer. We had met at the airport a year after my marriage ended. He asked me where I was from and laughed when I said I was English. He probed. 'You need to know you're black'. This was an important relationship for me in working on my identity. He was very angry about transracial adoptions and extremely articulate about most issues, but he was angry about my upbringing. 'It's just the white part of you that's bad' was the phrase he used to justify his violence towards me. I desperately wanted to keep my baby. He was determined that I would not. I was 'mixed race' and being the mother of his child would be unacceptable to his family. He threatened my life and the baby's life if I dared to go ahead against his wishes. I was terrified and had no self-confidence, and was also confused. He once told me I had a duty 'to breed the white blood out of me', that he was 'my saviour', had rescued me from my 'white life', and picked me up from the gutter. My self-esteem was very low when we met; it was rock bottom when we parted. Early in the relationship, I stored some of my belongings at his home. When I went to collect them I discovered he had thrown away most of my books and records. 'But they were white,' he said, 'your previous life'. I was shocked and devastated. They were books and records I had collected over twelve years, part of the work of building my identity. His became a crude and dangerous form of total cultural immersion.

I had just completed my first year at university and I was also working every evening in a law firm. I became suicidal, expecting to fail my exams although I did pass with good marks. Then I became deluded. I thought my adoptive mother was trying to kill me. I saw her at the wheel of every vehicle on the road, on the train and on the tube. My fear of her went back to the time when, as a pupil at the convent school, my mother was deeply resentful of me. Her father's sudden death when she was thirteen meant she was forced to leave school and work in a factory to support her mother and four younger siblings. Her hopes and dreams were shattered. In my state of madness, I believed she would punish me for getting another chance to study when a second chance was never an option for her.

I was admitted to a psychiatric ward in 1990. It was to be the first of many such stays when I suffered suicidal depression. I was told by a consultant that only medication would help, that I was aiming too high by attending university. Nurses told me I should have known better than to be with a South Asian man as 'they always beat up their wives'. This stereotyping silenced me. But the fourth psychiatrist I saw was a French woman married to an Indian with mixed race children. She immediately recommended psychotherapy for which I was so grateful. I wish I could thank her personally. She probably saved my life. Although I was readmitted to hospital during my studies, I remained in therapy for several years. In 1993 I graduated with an honours degree in law.

In hospital I witnessed persistent neglect, sexual harassment and abuse of women, people with physical impairments, lesbians and gay men. Adopted and fostered people are particularly vulnerable to abuse. Our experiences are often misunderstood and misinterpreted. My last psychiatric admission was in 1996. Concerns about my physical health were explained away as adverse effects of medication. A few months later I was diagnosed with relapsing remitting multiple sclerosis. I have no doubt that the chronic distress I have experienced has contributed substantially to my chronic physical illness. I became involved in the mental health system survivors movement and have worked with other black survivors and professionals to influence change in mental health services through education and training.

I'm still shocked by the entrenched racist beliefs of some social workers where I work in southern England. This is where so many transracial placements occur. Until I met transracially adopted people brought up in multiracial areas, I believed that some of the problems would be solved if white adoptive parents were prepared to move to those areas. But I have met many adopted and fostered adults brought up in London who are emotionally isolated and alienated from black cultural life.

A self-help group, the Association of Transracially Adopted and Fostered People was formed in 1993. It is here that I have received a lot of support from people with similar experiences to my own. Their presence in my life has enriched my life immeasurably. Mostly we remain silent about our feelings within our adoptive families, not wishing to hurt or to be disloyal to the people who have loved and nurtured us. Carefully concealing the pain of our culture being ignored or patronised, of feelings of not belonging, of unexpressed grief causes much distress. In 1998 I attended group counselling for transracially placed people at the Post-Adoption Centre. In 1999 I referred myself to an inter-cultural therapy centre. For two years the expertise of a black female psychotherapist enabled me to uncover so much internalised racism, helping me to understand and overcome feelings of low self-worth and self-loathing.

The emotional damage I sustained in childhood left me vulnerable to abuse. I was pathologised by psychiatric services as unable to sustain intimate relationships. Yet the underlying causes were not acknowledged; the experts implied that sustained relationships, however abusive, were acceptable. I now have a relationship of nearly five years with my partner. It is joyful, loving and respectful. He is white, English and has been deeply committed to fighting racism for many years. His commitment has been a critical factor in building the trust I need to function fully in a relationship.

My adoptive mother is 82 and my adoptive father is 85. When my father was admitted to hospital suddenly with an acute asthma attack, my mother was shocked and confused. My mother has a lymphoma and multi-infarct dementia. In her confusion, my mother told me that she was the adopted child in our family. I had to place her in temporary residential care while my father was away. The social worker, who had hardly spoken two words to my mother, then coerced my father into placing her in permanent residential care. But my father recovered and was determined to look after her at home and she, too, was determined to go home. I arranged a mental health advocate for her and for my father to be supported by his GP. We had to change the social worker. Now they are together again – at home. I know what it's like not to have a voice. My experiences enabled me to support them in this way. I needed to do that for them.

I hope one day to become a full-time writer. Some brilliant contemporary poets such as Jackie Kay who wrote *The adoption papers* have articulated the experience of transracial placement. Their creative use of language has inspired me to devote more time to finding my own voice through writing poetry and prose. Recently I received a Mind Millenium award to create and perform a collective poem with other transracially adopted and fostered poets.

My name Veronica means true image. My adoptive parents did not change my name; it was my birth mother's choice and, as a Catholic, I was brought up believing I was named after Saint Veronica. It was not a legacy I could sustain. I later learned that I was named after Veronica Lake, the Hollywood actress. Physically we could not be more different. I have taken many diversions in seeking my true image, like a human chameleon – a Zelig character. I have come to realise the importance of not changing to be acceptable to others, but to accept myself, however unacceptable that may be, and to allow the truth to emerge.

Adoption is dislocating and confusing. Loss is distressing and disorientating. Racism is devastating; it claims lives. Children, often vulnerable, chaotic, frightened and suicidal, need defenders, protectors, role models. Many adoptive parents do not acknowledge or understand the subtleties of racism. When challenged they become confused and defensive, or say it's not a problem for them, that the 'problem' lies with the child, their inherited genes, or with black people in general. The current government feels vindicated in condemning the harmful nature and complexity of racism in British society; an ill-informed electorate insisting that same race placements have 'gone too far'. Deliberately handing this legacy to innocent children when as adults we know how heavily racism weighs on us, is surely what has gone too far.

How can we best support black or mixed race adopted children so that their identities remain strong, positive and intact despite the reality of institutional racism? Why are these children continuing to be denied their right to grow up in a black or mixed race adoptive family? Where is the government's commitment to providing and resourcing comprehensive pre-adoption and post-adoption services that meet the needs, as defined by ourselves, of black and mixed race adopted children, birth relatives and adoptive parents?

Is anyone listening to our experiences? The silence has never been louder.

15

AVOIDING DISRUPTION
Concurrent planning

Gill Gray

Concurrent planning is an approach to permanency planning for children in the care system. Based on the work of Linda Katz (Katz *et al.*, 1994), this method has been pioneered over the last 20 years by the Lutheran Social Services in Seattle, yet remains very much in its infancy in the UK. With only three projects – in Manchester, Brighton and London – operating a concurrent planning scheme, there is still some way to go in terms of developing this exciting and challenging new approach to care planning for babies and very young children who are the subject of care proceedings.

The government has given attention to the plight of children in the care system through initiatives such as Quality Protects and the Adoption and Children Act, both of which have highlighted a range of problems faced by these children. Major concerns have been voiced about the number of placement changes that many such children have to endure and about the length of time that it can take for final decisions to be reached as to where, and with whom they should reside permanently. For the children involved these factors can have major implications. As we know from attachment theory and the work of David Howe (1998), children who have not had the opportunity during their very early lives to settle and form secure attachments with a primary carer, or who have had these attachments disrupted or broken, can continue to have difficulty in trusting people and in forming the strong and secure bonds with others that are so crucial to their future security and emotional health.

We also have increasing evidence of just how important environmental factors during the first year of life are for an infant's long- term cognitive and emotional development (Perry *et al.*, 1995). The government's concern that there should be no drift in planning and decision making for such young children is born out by this developing body of knowledge.

The aim of concurrent planning is to prevent these difficulties from occurring by avoiding unnecessary moves for the children involved and by ensuring that final decisions regarding their permanent care are made within their timescales. This is achieved by placing the children with concurrent planning carers who are approved not only as foster carers but also as potential adopters.

A child placed with concurrent planning carers is essentially fostered by them in the first instance while assessments of the birth family are undertaken as a part of the care proceedings. Regular contact with the birth family is supervised and takes place in a neutral setting. The carer's work, during this time, is to develop a positive relationship with the birth family, in which all parties are focused upon the best interests of the child. The two-way sharing of information about the child's likes and dislikes, health and development, history and so on, is encouraged.

Throughout the court proceedings staff from the concurrent planning team undertake the assessment work with the birth parents, and their extended families, and also support them. While this work is continuing a close watch is maintained on the court's timetabling of the case. The maximum length of time for a concurrent planning case to be processed through the court from the early stages to the final hearing aims to be no more than nine months.

If the court decides that a child should then return to the birth family, the concurrent planning carer's role will be to assist this move in a way which is focused on the child's needs, in order that the child's attachment to his or her carers is maintained. If, on the other hand, the plan agreed for the child is one of adoption outside of the birth family the concurrent planning carers will then apply to adopt the child themselves, thus avoiding the need for the child to be disrupted, or suffer a broken attachment with the person who has been his or her primary carer.

Situations considered suitable for concurrent planning are those in which it is anticipated from the outset that there is a 60–80 per cent chance that the child will not be able to be rehabilitated safely to their birth family following assessment. Typically, concurrent planning cases are those where birth parents have severe mental health problems or where they have chronic histories of alcohol or drug misuse, where previous rehabilitation attempts have failed, or situations where older siblings have been removed from the family as a result of any of these factors or as a result of severe neglect. While these family circumstances may be common to many children in the care system, the difference here is that from the outset there is the poor prognosis of the birth parents being able to resolve their difficulties within their child's timescale. Cases accepted for concurrent planning are, therefore, accepted on the basis that birth parents will be offered what is effectively a 'last chance' to overcome their problems.

Exponents of concurrent planning are keen to point out the advantages in this way of working. Most easily understood are, perhaps, the benefits for the child who will return to their birth family or go on to be adopted by their carers. In this way the child is in a situation which either way can only have a positive outcome; it is the adults involved who are expected to carry the risks and uncertainties on behalf of that child. Furthermore, by encouraging birth parents and concurrent planning carers to work together, it is hoped that the children who go on to be adopted will develop a much richer under- standing of their circumstances of their early life than may happen in traditional adoptions.

The benefit of concurrent planning for birth parents perhaps requires closer consideration. Given the principle that concurrent planning offers a 'last chance' for them it is essential that these parents receive the best possible opportunity to overcome their difficulties. In traditional care proceedings it is not unusual for birth parents to feel sidelined or left to deal with their problems alone, while social workers focus on the statutory needs of the child and the demands of the court proceedings. In concurrent planning birth parents are allocated their own worker who will support them in whichever way is appropriate. For some birth parents the realisation that this is indeed their last opportunity to regain care of their child will provide sufficient motivation for them to make full use of this opportunity.

It is not unusual for a sense of mutual understanding and respect to develop between the birth family and the concurrent planning carers. In some cases birth parents have been able to relinquish their child for adoption having developed a sense of trust in the carers. Decisions regarding the desira- bility of continuing contact after adoption with members of the birth family are more likely to be considered positively if, as in concurrent planning, all parties have a sense of what to expect from each other.

A question commonly asked, is what, if any, are the benefits of concurrent planning for the carers involved, given the stressful nature of what they are being asked to undertake and given, too, that there are more secure routes by which to adopt a child? For each concurrent planning carer there is perhaps a different motivational force at play. For some it is the opportunity to adopt a baby or very young child when most adopters are offered older children with more complex needs; for others it may be a desire to be involved in an extremely child-focused process which will benefit the child irrespective of the outcome. All such carers need to accept fully, however, that their role in the first instance is that of a foster carer with the aim of rehabilitation for the child with the birth family.

For all the perceived advantages, concurrent planning is not without its critics. There are those who remain opposed to it on the grounds that, in their eyes, the odds are stacked against the birth parents from the outset and that concurrent planning constitutes little more than a route to adoption by the back door. This argument overlooks the fact, however, that it is the court that determines, ultimately, whether cases are suitable for concurrent planning. As in all cases the court has a responsibility to ensure that the birth parents in concurrent planning case receive a fair hearing.

The Human Rights Act, 1998 has led some to question whether birth parents' rights are considered sufficiently, chiefly in relation to Article 8(1), the 'right to respect for . . . family life'. It is important to remember two points here: first, that birth parents in concurrent planning will have been identified from the outset as being at risk of losing custody of their children. Far from seeking to remove or interfere with their right, the concurrent planning is an attempt to salvage family life for the birth family. Second, the children involved also have a right to a family life: concurrent planning aims to maximise the chances of this being achieved on their behalf.

Other criticisms of concurrent planning have focused upon the dual roles of the concurrent planning projects in both assessing and supporting birth parents while also supplying the carers. How do project workers remain impartial in such circumstances? The answer lies in good staff support and supervision and in the practice of separate workers having differing roles and functions. In the writer's experience workers are more likely to become split in support of their respective clients rather than entering into a collusive relationship with one another at the expense of the birth parents.

One of the most contentious aspects of concurrent planning, however, lies within the area of contact between the child and the birth parents. Established practice has usually been for contact in these circumstances to be offered at as great a frequency as possible as anything less than this has been thought to be detrimental to the bonding process between the parents and child. In actual fact, as Quinton *et al.* (1997) found, there is no empirical evidence to show that a moderate, rather than more frequent level of contact, as offered in concurrent planning, bears any direct relation to the nature or strength of this bond. In concurrent planning contact between parents and their child is offered initially at a maximum of three times per week.

There are good reasons for this level of contact being set. All concurrent planning cases involve especially vulnerable babies and children, all of whom will have experienced one or more separations, and many of whom will have been born suffering from drug withdrawal symptoms, foetal alcohol syndrome or other such medical conditions. All require particularly calm and settled environments in order to thrive. Given the demands on these children during the care proceedings in terms of assessment and observation etc., a level of three times per week contact is seen to be a realistic balance to maintain their links with their birth parents, while at the same time ensuring that their overall needs are met. The level of contact in concurrent planning cases is, however, reviewed regularly and adjusted accordingly.

Concurrent planning actively encourages birth parents to devote their time and energies in the short term to addressing their own problems and acknowledges that most will be unable to do so adequately if expected to maintain a high level of contact with their child at the same time. For a birth parent struggling to overcome an addiction, for example, maintaining a high level of contact can be unrealistic. Far from being a punitive measure, this approach to contact is designed to be enabling and encouraging of birth parents.

Although concurrent planning originated in the United States, it does offer a method of working which is very much in line with current official thinking about adoption and the needs of children in the care system. Concurrent planning is an extremely child-centred process. There are evident advantages in this way of working for the children themselves, for their birth parents, and for the concurrent planning carers; nevertheless many professionals have yet to be convinced.

It is still too early to know just how concurrent planning will develop in United Kingdom, whether its remit will be extended and whether other similar projects will emerge. It will be several years before the results of research being undertaken are known. In the meantime, interest in this approach continues to grow and spark debate nationwide. The ultimate test of concurrent planning, however, will and should, of course, be determined by what it offers those children and families whom it is striving to help.

References

Department of Health (2000), *Adoption: a new approach*, London.

Howe, D. (1998), *Patterns of adoption: nature, nuture and psychosocial development*, Oxford, Blackwell.

Katz, L., Spoonermore, N. and Robinson, C. (1994), *Concurrent planning*, Lutheran Social Services of Washington and Idaho.

Perry, B. D., Pollard, R., Blakley, T. L., Baker, W. L. and Vigilante, D. (1995), Childhood trauma, the neuro-biology of adaptation and 'use-dependent' development of the brain: how 'states' became 'traits', *Infant Mental Health Journal*, vol. 16, no. 4, Winter.

Quinton, D., Rushton, A., Dance, D. and Mayes, D. (1997), Contact between children placed away from home and their birth parents: research issues and evidence, *Clinical Child Psychology and Psychiatry*, 2(3), pp. 393–413.

16

HOW POST-ADOPTION SUPPORT CAN MAKE ADOPTION A SUCCESS

Val Forrest

The making of an adoption order is not the end of the matter – adoption is a life-long experience. The benefits, joys and necessity of adoption are well documented but since loss is a central theme for all parties in adoption, and will undoubtedly surface and resurface at different stages, there is inevitably a strong likelihood that there will be a need for support, advice or information over time.

Post-adoption support has a crucial role to play in making the experience a positive one for all those involved, ideally acknowledging the need for families to get on with the business of being a family knowing that support is readily available. Children need, for example, to know about their origins, adoptive parents need to know how to open up the issue and birth parents need to know that all is well for the child they lost.

In response to the justifiable demands of those families and individuals in need of support, there is a growing professional awareness of the crucial role of support to sustain adoptions. The availability of post-adoption support can stimulate recruitment of prospective adoptive parents as well as prevent adoption breakdown. Twenty per cent of adoptions of older children fail because of the pressure on adoptive parents who are struggling with damaged children with no support.

Commitment to develop expertise and provide good quality post-adoption support services is affected by funding and resources in both the voluntary and statutory sector. Service provision has not been uniformly developed and has resulted piecemeal provision in one area next to well-resourced and highly organised services in a neighbouring agency. There are high expectations that in the forthcoming overhaul of adoption legislation heralded by the Adoption and Children Act, 2002 will place a clear and uniform duty on all adoption agencies to provide effective post-adoption support of the highest quality, underpinned by clear policy.

A good post-adoption support service that will really make a difference in practice and policy must:

- promote services positively, take a proactive approach, and remove the stigma too often experienced by those who ask for help;
- be accessible to black and minority ethnic groups – research into needs is mostly related to white British families which raises serious questions about access and appropriateness of services;
- respond promptly to requests for help from all parties;
- have an educative role; and
- identify support needs of all parties at the 'matching' stage.

Support is often offered case by case, not prioritised and with no clear post-adoption support policy to underpin work with all parties. At least a dedicated post and preferably a team of specialist workers are needed to respond adequately to the ever-increasing demand for post-adoption support. There is a greater need to recognise the importance of ethnicity, race, culture and religion in planning appropriate services to support black families, including transracial placements. The needs of adopted children with disabilities requires greater attention.

Birth parents are often marginalised – the feelings associated with the loss of a child through adoption persists throughout life and can seriously affect the mental health of some birth mothers. Their support needs must be acknowledged.

The minefield of issues to be navigated by people affected by adoption is likely to include indirect or direct contact between birth and adoptive family members, exploring identity, explaining about adoption, infertility, loss of child to adoption, educational problems, and relationship problems – for all parties.

The adoption of babies has reduced considerably since the 1970s. Children placed for adoption today – black and of mixed parentage and white children – are likely to be older, may be a sibling group or have disabilities. Combined with the increase in inter-country adoption as well as step-parent adoptions, the issues that all parties are grappling with are increasingly complex. Children who are older when placed for adoption are likely to have experienced serious family discord, disruption and fragmented attachments and possibly physical or sexual abuse. Although the debate around same-race placements brought to the fore the importance of race and identity in family placements, trans-racial placements devalue the importance of race and culture and disregard the heritage of black children. While such placements are decreasing, inter-country adoption is increasing and frequently involves the adoption of black children by white parents. Children adopted in this way not only lose their birth parents but their country and their culture in exchange for the nurture of a new family and a good material standard of living. It remains to be seen, whether or not a white British family can promote the psychological well-being of a black child. The need for support will be considerable.

Children's need to find out more, develop a better sense of identity, understand their history, and requests for information about medical history are often different ways of saying the same thing. The wish to link with the past seems always to be there simmering away under the surface and can have a serious effect on home life if ignored. It is short sighted and indeed potentially damaging for adoption agencies to disregard this warning. While there are excellent examples of good practice in local authority post-adoption support, work is largely with adult adoptees in line with the Adoption Act 1976. Staffing levels have remained at a minimum over the past 20 years and many authorities struggle to cover this work with one part-time worker. Indeed many voluntary agencies are rapidly overtaking statutory provision in responding to the need to offer early support and work with quite young children in their adoptive families, in recognition that adoptive placements are becoming ever more complex. Many local authorities are waiting to take the lead from forthcoming legislative changes. Hence direct work with children in their adoptive families is not currently given priority.

I have yet to come across a 'typical' referral – each situation is unique. There are of course some common threads that are useful to keep in mind in working with families who wish to explore links with birth family members (usually a birth mother). From the perspective of the adopted child, the following account looks at the way in which support may be woven in to the process leading to a reunion with a birth mother.

A limited amount of information may satisfy a young child's (six to seven years) need to know more to develop a clearer sense of themselves by gaining a fuller picture of origins. Life-story-book work may well achieve this. Children often express a very natural wish for more information about their birth mother when they are as young as nine or ten. This often develops into an active wish to trace and meet her. Supporting this work may span a prolonged period of time and it is not uncommon for six or seven years to have elapsed from the point of an initial enquiry to a face-to-face meeting. Not all adopted people wish to be reunited with a birth mother but for those who do, the wish doesn't goes away.

The response from adoptive parents about this need to know more is important. That it is taken seriously is crucial. At this point contact with post-adoption support services can make an important difference to adoptive parents who are struggling to protect their child and themselves. It brings to the fore all the pain of original losses. Their experience is outside the mainstream and not likely to be shared by many people in their network apart from other adoptive families who have had the same experience. They often feel torn between the need to protect their son or daughter and the wish to help them gain a more realistic and less idealised picture of their birth mother, to stop taking out the pain on their adoptive parents who are sitting with their own pain.

Contact between the adoptive family and post-adoption worker is important at this stage to develop a positive environment in which to offer support, to explore support needs, personal resources and an understanding of the complexity of the issues for themselves and the birth family.

Of course this contact visit is poignant and may at first seem enough and for some it is – for now. Eventually it might generate a need to know more. Depending upon the age and stage a child is at, it may be appropriate to help them to gain a clearer concept of their early life and a concrete sequence of events by creating a visual representation of events through a life map or time-line drawing. This gives a very concrete picture and can be enriched by including such details as time and weight at birth, who knew of the birth, who was present at the birth and so on. Careful thought needs to be given to this work as the 'story' may be very painful and may be difficult to come to terms with.

The pleasure, inherent tensions and competing support needs encountered by all parties during this emotional journey make the task very complex. The child's age, level of understanding, support from adoptive parents, as well as the likelihood of establishing contact with a birth relative will all play a crucial role. The intensive continuing support of a skilled and experienced worker in the field of post-adoption work is an essential ingredient.

It may be worth considering contacting people from the network involved at the time of adoption, taking photographs of the maternity hospital, nursery and so on. Gaps can be filled in and a different perception of the birth mother developed which can help to give a more rounded picture. The post-adoption worker is, in most instances, unlikely to be the person involved at the time of the adoption so will be working with second-hand information from the file.

Adolescence brings fresh challenges to the adoption scene. A child who has joined their family through adoption has usually, often unconsciously, developed a strategy to help them cope with major life changes but a change of school (for example, a move to secondary school) can be a fraught and frightening time. The difficult, acting-out behaviour, which frequently accompanies such times, is easily misconstrued and the significance of a child's growing sense of insecurity around identity is often missed. Of course not all difficult behaviour has its roots in adoption, but it is important that its relevance is explored. A referral for post-adoption support may come from the school, therapeutic services, or directly from an adoptive parent on behalf of their son or daughter.

Problems which may have manifested themselves at school in terms of disruptive or withdrawn behaviour, poor concentration, limited attainment, peer relationship problems, or strained relationships with siblings and parents – often with an adoptive mother – can develop from a child's growing need to know more about their origins. A complex process is involved in building a sound identity; it is perplexing and preoccupying especially during adolescence. Even with information available from adoptive parents, there remains a need to gain full information from 'official' sources. Whatever information an adopted person already has, it can feel doubly validating to see that same information with the post-adoption counsellor.

Seeking information is the first step in building a complete person – finding the missing pieces of the jigsaw or filling the hole that adopted children often refer to. This is especially so for black and mixed parentage children who have been separated from their black identity though transracial adoption.

As the child gets older, the need for a more sophisticated telling of their story is required – 'Your birth mum couldn't take care of you' might become 'Your birth mum was too ill to take care of you and you couldn't wait while she got better'. The wish to further explore their history and understand, at whatever level, why and what happened, can help build a more secure sense of identity.

Finding out about one's origins is likely to have a profound effect for most people, but for children this is particularly true. The younger the child the greater may be the need to slow the process down. Ideally one would wish an adopted person to have a well-developed sense of security before exploring the possibility of opening up contact with birth family members. And yet it is the gaps in the history that add to a sense of insecurity and may only be filled once contact is re-established. There will be a delicate balance for all involved – to get on with life and yet proceed knowing that the consequences of opening things up further could be disastrous. Sometimes there is a sense that 'we are coping so badly that the risk is worth taking in the hope that things move on'.

Children who are seeking information about their family of origin often have a number of issues at the fore and may well be receiving therapy. This work needs to be undertaken by a therapist with knowledge and experience of the psychology of adoption. It is not infrequent for the view held by those working in clinical or therapeutic services to conflict with the practice and philosophy of those involved in post-adoption work. It is often said that a child is emotionally too fragile or vulnerable to consider opening up the issue of contact with birth relatives. Of course it would be foolish to think this is never the case, but some crucial healing opportunities may be missed, if the child's need to know is not seen as central. There will always be the dilemma, is now the right time?

Once contact is opened up, don't go too far too soon. People are at their most vulnerable. Try to take small steps not big strides. Of course, the main source of support for a young adopted person is most likely to be their parents who, in turn, need support. Often they are instinctively doing the right thing but may well feel demoralised, despairing, powerless, angry and frustrated in varying degrees. Their sense of self-worth may be well and truly dented. Extra help is needed to support the adoptive parents to open up this topic;

they are not failing if they need help, it's a very hard task. There is a continuum of need and further face-to-face contact with the post-adoption counsellor can be helpful. Support gives everyone the chance to deal with the unexpected and to consider everyone's feelings.

It might be two or three months before the next contact is made by the family. There is a roller coaster effect with highs of elation and troughs of depression particularly if the story is distressing. It is vital that the family dictates the pace of this work, as they will need time to process information and their emotional reaction to it. They will come back when they are ready and feel strong enough to deal with the powerful emotions that are evoked. It is not likely that the birth parent 'in the shadow' will disappear. A child can be pressing hard to open up contact further without any current knowledge of the physical and mental health of the birth mother. He or she may well try to force a reunion, become so obsessed with the idea of meeting a birth mother to the exclusion of all else, even risking possible further rejection.

Providing old details such as an address is still relevant. A very carefully worded letter may be sent from the counsellor to the birth mother outlining the adopted person's wish for up to date information and to hear her version of events surrounding the adoption.

It is important that the post-adoption counsellor meets with the birth mother personally to seek her views. It is essential to explore thoroughly the implications of what is requested and her preparedness to undertake contact at this time as well her need for support. She may feel a sense of inadequacy, as well as considerable fears of being judged all over again. She may worry that she may not measure up to what her son or daughter is seeking. The post-adoption worker may fill in the gaps (if this has been agreed by the adoptive family) and say what has happened to her since the adoption.

The child may also wish to put in their own words what it is they are seeking. It may help to crystallise exactly what is going on for them. The pain of early rejection can begin to be explained by the birth mother. Adopted children need to hear from their birth mother that they were loved and wanted if only things had been different. It is important that the child does not feel responsible for what happened in the past nor feels that he or she must look after their birth mother in the future. Indeed a birth parent can play an important role in releasing her adopted child from the sense of responsibility to look after her.

The adoptive parents' need for support at this point will be heightened. They may feel left out and fear the loss of their child back to their birth family, a loss of control over the situation, a revival of the painful loss of infertility, and an overwhelming sense of vulnerability. The child, pulled in both directions, can feel omnipotent yet out of control, fear further rejection, and can be overwhelmed by a sense of responsibility for everybody.

An exchange of letters, news and photographs is generally agreed as the best way forward. Letters can be cathartic for all but far from easy to write. Some reality can be injected into the story: 'She wasn't ready to be a parent ... was too ill to look after a child ... she was ill and couldn't, and you couldn't wait'. It is important not to leave the child with regrets. But if the content is too emotional, this is likely to be reciprocated which can then come as a shock. If letters are non-committal, the response is likely to be the same which can feel disappointing. It helps to have something tangible: photographs are important – of the child as a baby, the birth mother, the birth mother and baby together, and of the adopted child.

The age of the child is likely to continue to determine next steps. In some situations there will be a continuing exchange of news and photographs perhaps twice a year using a letterbox service often managed by the post-adoption counsellor whereby addresses and adoptive surnames can be kept confidential. Most agencies use a contract to set this up. Choosing when to exchange may seem like a minor detail that is often overlooked but so frequently families comment that birthdays are too painful a time to choose, as they serve as a very painful reminder to all. Each individual will have their own view of when it is best for them. Using a contract to record the frequency and time of exchanges gives them structure and clarity. It can be reassuring to have a clear boundary and sense of what to expect from each other. Contracts do not need to be rigid and can be renegotiated in line with everyone's changing needs.

The key players ultimately determine decisions about face-to-face contact. There is probably no obvious *right* time. The key point is that good support for all parties must continue to be part of the process. The counsellor will offer support to explore everyone's preparedness for reunion and be available through the process in whatever way is most helpful.

While meeting a birth mother does not remove a sense of conflict for the adopted child, it can allow them to leave the anger and pain of rejection behind and really move on. There is the potential to heal old wounds that enable both the birth and adoptive parents to gain a sense that they have 'got their child back'. It can make a big difference to family relationships but most of all, once the euphoria has subsided, it can give way to a renewed and solid sense of identity for the adopted child.

17

TALKING AND TELLING

Julia Feast and David Howe

Over the last 50 years we have learned a great deal about the needs of children who are separated from their family at birth. We appreciate how important it is for children to have access to information about themselves, so that they might better understand who they are, and begin to develop a clear sense of identity. Communicating factual information about family history is seen as an integral part of this process. For the adoptive parent this can be a challenging and sometimes difficult task. Giving and receiving information about complex and sensitive matters, and dealing with children's reactions and responses require great skill.

Research and practice experience remind professionals about the importance of adoptive parents communicating clearly and openly when talking about adoption and children's origins. Good communication is critical if children are to grow up with a strong sense of identity, and a clear understanding of who they are and what makes them tick. Adoptive parents are encouraged to talk openly with their children about their adoption, origins and previous experiences. However, in cases where birth parents have been involved in sexual or physical abuse, inflicted emotional neglect, abused drugs or alcohol, or have been victims of rape or incest, the process of telling and discussion is rarely easy or straightforward.

Professionals are charged with the responsibility of preparing prospective adoptive parents for the task of telling. Parents have to be helped to develop the knowledge, understanding, skills and confidence needed to handle the discussion. In theory, we know that being open and frank provides opportunities for the child to acquire information and gain confidence in asking questions about origins, but in practice it can be a difficult and anxious experience. When both parent and child feel anxious and sense the mutual unease that the subject provokes, the topic is first avoided and then ignored. Often, parents may conclude: If my child seems happy and is not asking questions, then why raise the subject?

The authors recently completed a study that compared the characteristics and experience of 394 adult adopted people who searched for birth relatives (searchers) with 78 adult adopted people who had not searched but whose birth relatives had made an enquiry about them (non-searchers) (Howe and Feast, 2000). Although 40 per cent of adopted people in the study acknowledged that their parents had been willing in principle to discuss the adoption and its background, only 29 per cent said that they had felt entirely comfortable raising the topic with them. Half of all respondents said they felt satisfied with the level of information about their adoption given to them by their parents, leaving the remaining half either unsure (21 per cent) or dissatisfied (29 per cent) with the amount of knowledge available or revealed.

The majority of both searchers and non-searchers said they had thought about their birth family while growing up. For example, 85 per cent of all adopted people said they had wondered what their birth relatives, particularly their birth mother, looked like and whether they looked like them. Sixty-six per cent also wondered why they had been placed for adoption. For most, these thoughts remained private and were not shared with their adoptive parents. In part this was because there was a wish not to worry their parents, and in part it was a subject that they felt was intrinsically difficult and awkward. Some people feared that asking questions about their background would be interpreted as being dissatisfied with their adoption. It is, therefore, important for adoptive parents to realise that an absence of questions does not necessarily mean that the adopted person is not interested in receiving knowledge.

The study investigated the experience of people, the majority of whom were adopted before the Children Act, 1975. It might therefore be argued that difficulties communicating information about a child's adoption might be an old issue, no longer relevant to today's world in which relatively few babies are placed. However, closer analysis of the findings suggests that older placed children were, in fact, *more likely* to have found the whole issue of talking and telling even more difficult than adopted people who had been placed as babies. For example, although 47 per cent of those placed *before* their third birthday said they felt uncomfortable asking for information about their adoption, this figure rose to 71 per cent for those placed *after* the age of three.

Similar findings are reported for other elements of the 'talking and telling' process. Of those placed under the age of three years, 43 per cent said that their adoption was openly discussed compared to only 18 per cent of those adopted older than the age of three. Fifty-three per cent who joined their adoptive parents before their third birthday expressed satisfaction with the level of information given about their adoption, a figure which fell to only 29 per cent for those placed beyond the age of three.

Equally interesting, those who felt that adoption was a relatively open and comfortable topic to raise with their adoptive parents and who expressed satisfaction with the level of information provided were much more likely to evaluate their adoption overall as a positive experience (also see Raynor, 1980, who reports similar findings). For example, 77 per cent of those who felt comfortable asking their parents for information evaluated their adoption as a positive experience. In contrast, of those who said that they felt uncomfortable asking their parents for information, only 44 per cent evaluated their adoption positively. A similar picture arises for whether or not the individual felt their adoption was openly discussed. Seventy-four per cent who said their adoption was openly discussed evaluated their adoption as a positive experience compared to only 38 per cent of those who felt that their adoption was not a subject for open conversation. Of course, it is appreciated that there is possibly a problem interpreting the direction of causal order here. Nevertheless it does appear that the issue of how well parents discuss and handle the subject of their child's adoption affects or is affected by the adopted person's evaluation of their overall experience of being adopted.

Along similar lines, a Department of Health funded initiative, Project 16–18 (Hundleby and Slade, 1999) consulted 58 adopted people aged 14–21. This study also revealed that in general adopted people still found talking about their early history with their adoptive parents difficult and problematic. Talk Adoption, a national freephone for adopted people under the age of 25 years old, received over 3,000 enquiries between 1997–9. The analysis of the service showed that a significant number of enquiries were received from adopted people who reported difficulties and feeling uncomfortable talking about their origins to their adoptive parents (Greenwood and Forster, 2000).

The findings of these two studies indicate that talking and telling continue to be an issue for adoptive parents and their children. Perhaps the fact that many of the children adopted today were in the public care system as a result of parental neglect, abuse or rejection makes 'telling' a particularly difficult task for adoptive parents. Relating information that may remind children about unhappy experiences can be unsettling and distressing for both the child and adult. It is, therefore, understandable why some adoptive parents feel hesitant about encouraging their child to seek information about their history, or avoid cues from the child hinting that perhaps they would like more information or discussion.

For example consider the case of Anthony. He was placed for adoption at the age of five. Until that time he had lived with his birth mother Denise and two older siblings and one younger sibling. None of the children's fathers were on the scene. When Anthony was born Denise told the health visitor that she had not wanted him and didn't feel motherly towards him. Anthony was physically well cared for, but there were concerns about his emotional health. He was very withdrawn and, other than with his siblings, he found it difficult to form relationships with other children of his age. Without any warning Denise took Anthony to the social services department on Christmas Eve and left him there. She told the social worker in the presence of Anthony that she did not like him and believed that there must have been some switch at birth. Anthony was clearly distressed but as the months went by and he settled with his adoptive parents he seemed recovered and happier. The adoptive parents had always thought it was important to talk to any child they adopted about his or her origins, but they found it too painful to remind Anthony of the circumstances of his adoption and the siblings he had left behind.

Raynor (1980) found that parents' ability to talk about adoption affected how well they 'told' their child about being adopted. Although many adopted people felt that their parents were uncomfortable discussing adoption, even amongst those seen as well-adjusted, levels of impaired psycho-social functioning increased if the adopted person reported that their parents seemed ill-at-ease talking about the adoption (Raynor, 1980). In Raynor's study a surprising 60 per cent of adopters said that they had kept back some information about the adoption from their child. Many adopters felt anxious, even insecure when discussing adoption with their adolescent child, even if their relationship was good. Parents said they felt worried that open discussion might threaten the child's sense of belonging.

If children sense that the subject of adoption makes their parents feel anxious, they may inhibit any mention of matters that carry an emotional charge. Anxiety in parents causes anxiety in children who may fear a second 'rejection' (Howe, 1998). Difficulties in dealing with relevant but potentially uncomfortable information may distort relationships and interfere with the ability of adopted children to develop a clear, confident and relaxed sense of their own identity.

Kirk (1964, 1981) was aware that a key task for the adopted child and his/her parents to handle was the issue of difference. Being adopted was felt to be an important and relevant difference that had to be acknowledged and addressed by adoptive parents. Kirk believed that adopters who did not acknowledge the difference – who 'rejected' difference – were denying a relevant and potentially important aspect of their child's origins and identity. Rejection of difference frustrates opportunities for the child to discuss a topic of central importance to their sense of identity and worth. Difference might receive a negative connotation if it cannot be talked about or acknowledged.

In contrast, parents who could comfortably 'acknowledge difference' were able to relate more honestly and openly with their children which served both parties well in terms of their long term adjustment and psychosocial development. Information was neither denied nor distorted. This allows adopters to empathise with their child. Empathy and good, open communication maximise the child's positive acceptance and understanding of who they are. Adopted children have to feel secure enough to differ from their adoptive parents and for this difference not to be perceived as threatening.

Adopters who are relaxed about the subject of adoption appear able to empathise with their child. Adopted adults in Raynor's (1980) study felt more satisfied if they thought their parents accepted their children's background. Children who believed that their parents were critical or disapproving of their birth parents were more likely to evaluate their adoption negatively. Raynor also observed that adopted people appeared better adjusted if their parents had met their birth parents. This early observation has important implications for current trends towards encouraging many adopted children to retain contact with their birth family, either directly or indirectly (also see Grotevant and McRoy, 1998; Neil, 2000).

Although at first sight appearing somewhat paradoxical, acknowledgement of adoption as a relevant autobiographical difference is, in fact, accepting and integrative (Howe, 1998). The resolution of the potential tension between acknowledgement of difference and integration and the promotion of feelings of belonging is a test of the parents' ability to handle the complex nature of parent–child relationships implied in adoption. However, Brodzinsky (1987) also warned against over-doing acknowledging the child's adoptive status – an approach he termed 'insisting on difference', which he felt was as damaging as rejecting difference.

Preparation and training for prospective adoptive parents has improved significantly over the years. Nevertheless, many adopted people continue to report feeling uncomfortable talking with their adoptive parents about their background. We need therefore to give more attention to the 'talking and telling 'process so that adopted people receive the information which they feel they need. Again and again, research studies suggest that most adopted children benefit from having as much information as possible about their genealogy, reason for being adopted, and their cultural, racial and ethnic heritage. The provision of such information is thought to be closely linked with the formation of a secure identity and feelings of self-worth.

Telling can never be a one-off event. It should be seen as part of the life cycle, evolving as the child's level of understanding increases and different questions are raised. Information at the time of the child's placement may need adding to, or new information may become available, for example the death of a birth parent. Adoptive parents may be presented with a dilemma about whether or not such information should be passed on to the child now or at a later stage of maturity and understanding.

Triseliotis et al. (1997) discuss direct work with adopted children. They recognise the majority of currently placed children have histories of hurt and adversity, matters which both children and their adoptive parents will need to face. Among the themes and issues the authors feel that parents and children need to consider include helping children deal with change and trauma, identity needs, and the creation and therapeutic value of life story books. Each of these might raise strong and possibly unresolved feelings in the child that will require sensitive handling by parents who in turn might require expert support, assistance and advice.

There is a need to assess and address the ability of prospective adoptive parents to talk openly and easily about sensitive and complex information, including facts about their child as well as their own feelings and experiences of loss and identity (for example, infertility). There is also a need to understand the child's perspective. This can help identify where support might be needed to facilitate communication between the child and his or her adoptive parents. For example, some children might not feel comfortable talking formally or face to face about matters which may be hard, upsetting or puzzling. Perhaps talking on a car journey is easier when children are sitting in the back seat behind their parents, or in the case of older children sitting in the front seats side by side. Some children may never feel really comfortable talking about their birth relatives with their adoptive parents. In these cases it may be appropriate to leave the child's life story-book in an accessible and familiar place such as a bedroom where it can be read in private. Adoptive parents might also want to let their child know where papers relating to their adoption can be found. This gives the child permission to browse their 'story' whenever they want.

Agencies and their practitioners should compile a portfolio of ideas, research findings and practice guidance upon which both professionals and parents might draw. Such resources provide a range of things to think about as well as various practical ideas to help identify needs and facilitate the communication process. The resource pack might include the following facts, ideas and practical suggestions:

- Make age-appropriate books, magazine and newspaper articles available to the adopted person.
- Story telling – use fictitonal characters to relate the experiences of the adopted child to stimulate dialogue and discussion.
- Play-use of art materials, dolls or role play to give children an appropriate medium in which to explore and express their thoughts and feelings.
- Acknowledge that it is natural to have questions and let children know that you are willing to answer all that you can.
- Make appropriately positive comments about the birth family so that the adopted child has a sense that the birth family (but not what they did if maltreatment is part of the history) is accepted by the adoptive family.
- Lay down knowledge and the whereabouts of significant people who might be willing to be contacted as sources of information about the child's early life.
- Provide information leaflets containing advice about the talking and telling process.
- Sensitise teachers, doctors, and other family and health core professionals to adoption issues helping them to regard as normal adopted people's interest and questions about their birth family.
- Make visits to the adopted child's area of origin.

There is a need to provide adoptive parents with opportunities to share difficulties they may be experiencing in trying to communicate with their child about his or her adoption. For example, an annual contact by the adoption agency either by personal visit, telephone call or letter with questionnaire can be offered which provides the chance for adoptive parents to report what is going well as well as share potential difficulties. Workshops or meetings for adoptive parents to come together and share experiences and learn from one another might be provided. Offering young adopted people the chance to join together, giving them the opportunity to discuss among themselves feelings they have about their adoption, including communicating with their parents is vital.

Children placed for adoption today are more likely to be older. Many have histories of neglect, abuse and rejection. Some will have either direct or indirect contact with their birth family. Nevertheless, talking and telling children about their adoption remain just as important as they were when adoption meant the placement of babies. In fact, the research evidence suggests that talk and discussion are both more important and more difficult with older placed children. The reasons for this are complex, based partly on the difficulties associated with talking about matters such as abuse and neglect, and partly to do with problems associated with establishing secure and open relationships with children whose emotional development may have been disturbed and upset in the years prior to their placement. Good preparation and continued post-adoption support are vital if parents are to build on their skills and sensitivities, maintain and develop an empathy with their children and birth families, and to keep open channels of communication that are clear and responsive.

References

Brodzinsky, D. (1987), Adjustment to adoption: a psychosocial perspective, *Clinical Psychological Review*, 7, 25–47.

Greenwood, S. and Forster, S. (2000), *Tell me who I am – young people talk about adoption,* Manchester, TALKadoption.

Grotevant, H. and McRoy, R. (1998), *Openness in adoption: exploring family connections*, Thousand Oaks, Sage.

Howe, D. (1998), *Patterns of adoption: nature, nurture and psycho-social development*, Oxford, Blackwell Science.

—— and Feast, J. (2000), *Adoption, search and reunion: the long term experience of adopted adults*, London, The Children's Society.

Hundleby, M. and Slade, J. (1999), *Project 16–18*, Nottingham, Catholic Children's Society.

Kirk, H. D. (1964), *Shared fate: a theory of adoption and mental health*, New York, Free Press.

Kirk, H. D. (1981), *Adoptive kinship*, Toronto, Butterworth.

Neil, E. (2000), The reasons why young children are placed for adoption: findings from a recently placed sample and implications for future identity issues, *Child and Family Social Work*, 5(4), 303–16.

Raynor, L. (1980), *The adopted child comes of age*, London, Allen & Unwin.
Triseliotis, J., Shireman, J. and Hundleby, M. (1997), *Adoption: theory, policy and practice*, London, Cassell.

18

KEEPING IN TOUCH

A different way of looking at post-adoption contact issues

Pam Hodgkins

When adoption in England and Wales was legalised in 1926, there were two key aims. The first was to get rid of the stigma of illegitimacy and the second was to protect the investment of the substitute parents. Seventy-five years later, this seems unbelievably outdated, yet the myth of adoption as a 'new start' or 'a clean sheet' pervades our practice, our thinking and probably our expectations. Why is this when we know that each one of us is today the sum of every experience and reaction we have experienced to date? Why do we not realise that we need to accommodate and reconcile the past within our hopes and plans for the future? If we can recognise this for ourselves and our families then we may well be on the road to recognising this fundamental truth for our work in adoption.

Adoption will only affect a small proportion of all children in coming years, a much smaller percentage than in the peak years of the 1960s, when babies were commonly placed. Many children, probably a majority, will experience some disruption of family life and deviation from a rose-tinted view of the two-parent nuclear family. Perhaps adoption workers should work with, and learn from leaders within the emerging network of child bereavement charities and those who support and advise stepfamilies as there will be much shared experience between all these types of family. In recognition of these enormous changes, the West Midlands Post-Adoption Service has taken a long hard look at the emotive issue of post-adoption contact and developed our own new approach.

We began by asking what those most closely involved were saying. We asked what we had learned in the past 25 years from the experience of adopted adults, in particular those who have exercised their right to seek their birth parents provided by the Adoption Act 1976. We reflected on what adoptive parents had told us both in times of joy and while in enormous difficulty. We listened to birth relatives, not only women who parted with babies for adoption because social pressures made it so difficult to be a single parent, but also to brothers, sisters, fathers and grandparents of those babies. We also listened to whole families who have more recently lost children to adoption through the care system either with their reluctant acceptance or in the face of their vigorous opposition. Adopted young people shared their experiences of being adopted, of engaging in various forms of 'contact', of a lack of 'contact' and in some cases, sadly, of the impact of disruption of their adoption upon their life.

We recognised that our gathering of information was not methodologically sound research, it was not clinical or quantitative but we considered that the very fact it came to us from so many diverse routes gave it an authenticity that should not be discounted. We have since found that more structured research as reported in *Adoption search and reunion* (Howe and Feast, 2000) and the first report of the longitudinal 'Contact after Adoption' study have reinforced our experience and soundings. As a group of experienced workers from a number of professional backgrounds linked by pragmatic attitude to problem solving and problem avoidance for all participants in adoption we began to develop a new approach. Our starting point was to look at modern family life in Britain. We asked some key questions and the answers made us wonder what was the intellectual basis for much of the work on post-adoption contact.

Our first discovery was that few colleagues could remember when they last wrote a letter that was not on a printed letterhead! Whilst only a few years ago people were writing weekly, monthly or annual letters to friends and relatives, this has been replaced by frequent phone calls. Low off peak charges as a result of competition in the telecommunications industry has resulted in the lengthy evening conversations with friends and relatives both in the UK and abroad with cost hardly a consideration. In fact the only relative common written communication among friends and family is the round robin Christmas communication that circulates widely amongst the middle classes with easy access to photocopiers or word processors. We are told that adult literacy standards are still declining and the old certainties that those who went to school would leave able to read write and count, even if science, geography and quadratic equations never touched their curriculum, are gone. We know that the families who most commonly lose children to adoption are from the sections of the community least likely to benefit from education. We are all aware that letters we know we should write fail to be written because we cannot find the right words. We do not write a letter of condolence but instead send a sympathy card with half a dozen words added in our own hand. We all know all this and yet one of the biggest growth areas in adoption practice in the past 20 years has been in 'postbox contact'. So we expect the least intellectually able to be able to communicate in the most challenging medium on the most emotive of subjects into the most abstract of settings. Is this really the most effective social work practice we can offer?

We also thought about the way in which our family life evolves. We move home, job, school and college far more frequently than in the past. We leave old communities and neighbours behind and embrace new ones but rarely with any intention of achieving a 'clean break'. We promise to 'keep in touch' both as security for ourselves in a time of change and uncertainty and to reassure those who are saddened by our departure. We rarely completely fulfil our promises and as the faces and names of those who once formed our day-to-day acquaintances pass across our mind we are filled with a mixture of regret and relief. We learn that keeping in touch needs commitment and some prioritising.

When we look at our activities and the groups we join we find constant evolution there too. A family may choose self-catering accommodation in a seaside location for the traditional bucket and spade holiday with pre-school children. The adventure of camping or caravanning may well be the favoured choice when the kids are of primary school age. Teenagers present a new challenge when everything that involves parents is boring. Eventually the opportunity may come for the parents to escape to the hotel they always dreamed of and try to relax while plagued by fears that their home may not be quite as they left it when they return. In 15 to 20 years, change has occurred resulting in no commonality between then and now. But what if the family was committed to returning to the same seaside bungalow for the same two weeks self-catering in the quiet resort with buckets and spades thrown in? Would the parents and teenagers look forward to it with equal commitment and enthusiasm as in the beginning? Not a chance! We know this but nevertheless we still make post-adoption contact arrangements which at least appear set in stone.

When thinking about the day-to-day activity of being a parent one can spot the evolution here too. The pre-school child goes wherever the parent chooses. Any physical resistance is overcome by using the backpack carrier, buggy or firmly held hand. Emotional resistance is resolved by bribery, incentives, threats or reasoning depending upon the style of parenting. A primary school age child does have a greater influence. There will be the commitment to fixed and fluid schedules of after school activities, socialising with friends, sports clubs, swimming lessons not to mention the not-to-be-missed vital television programmes. The teenager rarely has this problem. The parent's agenda does not feature in the wish list of the average teenager. The overriding principle appears to be if a parent suggests it an effective teenager will think of at least ten reasons why it is impossible, embarrassing or both. Once the child has grown into an adult the parent is no longer responsible for what the 'child' chooses to do or to leave undone; at that stage they simply have to cope with the comments and embarrassment that may result from those choices. Again we know and recognise all this yet we will still expect birth and adoptive parents to enter into agreements about post-adoption contact, which clearly fail to recognise this evolution at all. Should we ask ourselves if it is professional to bind people into agreements we know are destined to fail?

Finally, we asked ourselves what if we did not like, trust or respect certain relatives? Did we gain anything by keeping in touch with them? We concluded that every family probably had a relative that we called 'Auntie Lil'. 'Auntie Lils' are typically from a different social background and we often try to write them off as not 'real' relatives but 'in laws' or 'distant'. They will annoy us by their unreliability or their punctilious reliability. They fail to send gifts or embarrass us presenting us with unexpected or extravagant gifts when we are unable to reciprocate. We are unsure of their place in the family hierarchy and become irrationally jealous when someone close to us expresses closeness to or affection for an 'Auntie Lil'. When we plan significant family events we agonise over whether we need to invite 'Auntie Lil'. If we do we worry about what she may say or do and if we don't we fail to fully enjoy the event because we are feeling guilty about not inviting her. We can all recognise that 'Auntie Lil' puts us in a 'no win' situation. Whether 'Auntie Lil' wins or loses seems immaterial, whether 'Auntie Lil' is in the foreground or 'Auntie Lil' is in the shadows we will inevitably lose. We concluded that the birth relatives are potentially the 'Auntie Lils' of the adopter's family life and the adoptive parents are the potential 'Auntie Lil' in the birth family perspective.

Every family has its own dynamics and dilemmas. Families created by adoption will share many issues and each one will have those that are exclusively their own. The most common issue is that of loss. Loss permeates adoption, adopted children have lost birth parents as primary carers and adopted adults frequently report that with the loss of the birth parents went also a part of self and loss of identity. Traditionally they have also lost a whole extended family of birth relatives that may include grandparents and siblings. When the child leaves the birth family that family continues to change and the adopted child and adult into whom the child grows loses also a part of their future, the siblings and cousins born into the family after they left. Birth parents lose their child, they lose their hope for the future that was vested in that child. They live with an unfocused grief, one that has no specific time or place for the life of the child goes on although the life shared by the birth parent has ended. Like every parent who has lost a child they are angry, depressed, reproachful of others and of self. The knowledge that someone else may succeed in being a good parent to that child while they have failed is very hard to accept. Like in many difficult situations over a period of time the child is not talked of, embarrassed silence takes the place of tears and reproaches. The parents may move on into new relationships, new partners may know nothing of the adoption. If it was not a shared experience being helpfully empathetic may be too much of a challenge. Where the adoption was closed people may well feel powerless to achieve anything to help their partner, parent, son or daughter and so the 'least said soonest mended' philosophy provides a useful fallback position. A belief that nothing can be done leads to a situation where nothing is done through fear that doing something may cause an upset while doing nothing is acceptable.

Some people do not instantly recognise the losses experienced by the adoptive family. Adopters may still be grieving for the child they may have parented had they not experienced infertility or catastrophic pregnancies. They will at times feel keenly the sense of loss of that part of their child's life they did not share regardless of whether that amounted to days, months or years. They may be aggrieved by their loss of ability to be 'normal'; to be parents without the assessment of social workers, the medical adviser and the lawyers. However, adopters are supposed to be happy for they have adopted their child; the loss and grieving will have to be concealed.

So what if we acknowledge the loss, provide bereavement counselling and encourage everyone to get on with their lives in a 'normal' way? Will this create an acceptable normality in birth and adoptive families? It could be said that we tried variations of that way for the first 50 years of adoption history. It did not work. It is not possible to resolve the grieving process if the person grieved remains potentially able to be restored to the one who is grieving. The likelihood of repeating the early stages of the grieving process, the denial, the anger and the depression, are great. Becoming stuck in the depressive stage for years or decades is not exceptional.

The other factor which prevents adoptive and birth families from achieving the sense of normality most crave is a fear of causing any hurt or distress. There is no correlation between the extent to which adopted children talk to their adoptive parents about their birth families and the extent which they think, or are preoccupied by thoughts, of their birth family. Nothing is said but they sense it may cause upset or tension so they keep quiet. Adoptive parents shy away from pushing the birth parent issue because they do not want to upset the child. They may also find it more difficult to talk about the birth parents than they ever imagined. Teenage girls may talk to everyone outside their family, while teenage boys don't talk – they may kick the door or cat and ride off with reckless abandon at high speed on skateboard, bike, or motorbike. This subject is not one for day-to-day use, it only comes up at the most inappropriate times, particularly in the middle of an argument that appeared to be about something else altogether.

At the West Midlands Post-Adoption Service, we have learned most from groups when our service users have shared with other people affected by adoption what they wish they had been able to say and do if they had not been so inhibited by fear of hurting someone else. It is this fear of getting things wrong that inhibits people from trying to get it right. Perhaps it is fear of what could go wrong with direct contact that sways the vast majority of workers into favouring the ubiquitous letterbox contact. Are they trying to convince themselves that it is anymore possible to have indirect contact without consequences than it would be to have direct contact or no contact?

We decided we would strive to achieve a bespoke normality achieved through a sense of acceptance and reality that was comfortable for the family we were working with at that point in time, in the circumstances they found themselves. For our model, the family unit comprised those members of the adoptive family and the birth family who choose to become involved. We started by addressing what scared people. Adopters wanted to protect their children from the horrors of previous abuse, neglect and distress. They did not want the reality of that past invading their future. We could not collude with that, they had to face facts. The child they wanted to protect was there, you can't get more involved than that. Adopters are afraid that they will be unable to contain their own anger towards people who perpetrated such wrongs upon the child, or allowed such wrongs to occur.

We asked if they despised their child's birth parents? While children are glad to have a champion, someone they can be confident will protect them from harm they will soon become aware of the implications that they are not genetically related to those who protect them but are related to the perpetrators, the people despised by their protectors. The children may soon question whether the adopters despise not only the birth parents but also those characteristics and traits that the children have inherited from those parents. Those people the adopters may find so despicable are the very people who created the child the adopters claim to love unconditionally. There are ghosts to be laid here. How can we help adopters to convince their children that while they despise the wrongs that were done to the children, they do not despise the individual who did those things. Hate the sin, love the sinner is a useful shorthand. We also encourage adopters to develop empathy for the situation of the birth parents. We tell them of the Canadian proverb, 'Walk a mile in my moccasins to learn where they pinch', and question whether any of us would really prove ourselves good enough parents if we shared the history and circumstances of many birth families.

Adopters are also afraid of rocking the boat. If things are swimming along smoothly who needs the big C coming along and stirring everything up? If things are difficult and relationships fragile, well anyone can see that 'it's not a good time to even mention contact'. We are very close to not communicating.

Birth family members also experience fear of rocking the boat. If they have any means of communicating directly or indirectly with the adoptive family, they may not feel able to risk suggesting it could change, because to suggest change may result in less rather than more or nothing instead of very little. They say or write only the most bland and inoffensive words for fear that to use any expression of emotion would open the floodgates and they would never stop or to do so may cause offence. The result is communication that appears cool and indifferent. It is also unbelievably difficult to communicate effectively with someone you do not know.

Despite all these inherent difficulties, adopted children today are telling us they want more opportunities for contact with their birth families. Adult adopted people reinforce this by telling us of their day dreams and night-mares, in childhood and adolescence, about their birth relatives borne out of a complete lack of any communication. They tell us how difficult it can be to re-engage with a birth family in adulthood. How shared genes make you feel at home while lack of a shared history makes you feel an outsider. The international conference on adoption in 1991 in Edinburgh heard about a boy adopted from Korea, who was brought up in Sweden. He had told the researcher that despite the success of his adoption by every measurable indi-cator, he found that 'In Korea I feel Swedish, in Sweden I feel Korean!' Those poignant words sum up the experience of adoption. More children are coming to adoption from backgrounds where mental ill health and addiction to drugs and/or alcohol have taken their toll. They are bringing into their adoption explicit or hidden fears of what may happen to their birth parents when they are not there to look after them. On the one hand adopters want to protect their children from the awful reality of the circumstances of the birth parents, but this is like expecting their child to believe in Father Christmas when they are aged 12, a nice pretence but everyone knows it's not true. They need to show their strength in coping with the reality as a model for the children. If the worst should happen and the birth parents be critically ill or die, the child, of whatever age, will need the strength and support of the adopters to face that reality, to say a permanent goodbye, to grieve and to move on. This is far easier to achieve if the birth and adoptive families have never lost touch.

So how do we achieve and support a keeping in touch which is acceptable to everyone involved? We start with a presumption of openness rooted in confidence in the strength of the human spirit and the hope of doing better for the next generation. We reflect upon the reality that the two families are uniquely connected for life and expect all the adults involved to accept the responsibilities they have to one another and especially to any children involved. We cannot change history, amend legal orders, rewrite files. We have to start where we find ourselves today and focus on the future not the past. We have found it very helpful to build a link between two key players before directly engaging anyone else. The two mothers are often a great starting point as they have something in common – concern for the well being of the child that both could describe as 'my child'. They encounter each other with fear and trepidation. The adoptive mother assumes the birth mother will despise her because she has got her child. They need reassurance that the birth parents, anger was directed at the local authority. Resentment of the system can co-exist with acceptance of the adopters. The birth mother fears the adoptive mother will despise her for what she did or what she failed to do in the past. Our role is to help them overcome their fear. They need to recognise what each has given to the child and the role each may have in the future. What unites them is desire for the very best for their child. Adopters love to talk about their children, birth parents love to hear about their children. This is the first step in developing communication.

It can come as a very pleasant surprise to adopters to find that their child's birth parent is not quite the person they had visualised from their reading of a Form E or court report. Faced with the question 'What would I do if she turned up on my doorstep?' no longer provokes the panic, slam the door or move reaction but a far more manageable determination to put the kettle on. The realisation that both are equally scared and afraid of doing anything wrong helps. Whilst the adoptive mother is no longer scared witless by the prospect of the child disclosing his address, the birth parent would not want to risk this glimmer of light being snuffed out and would no more turn up on the adopter's doorstep than fly. They appreciate each other's position. They have a relationship and this makes it safe for the adopted child or adult to acknowledge his relationship to them both. Once two key people are reconciled they will draw in the other people who need to be involved.

We then need to sort out practicalities. How are they to keep in touch with each other? Do they want social work involvement? Would they prefer to be able to contact one another directly? If they want addresses to remain confidential, and it may well be many years before the myth of secrecy and confidentiality in adoption is finally laid to rest, then communication by e-mail may be the effective quick and easy option. This will depend on everyone having easy access to e-mail but now e-mail is available, with interactive TV as well as through computers, access will be much wider and could be achieved with a small grant if necessary. An e-mail address has the benefit of being infinitely transportable. Telephone contact, especially mobile phones, are another possibility but many people change their number with frustrating regularity and everyone needs to acknowledge that batteries may be flat or people unavailable to talk without any malicious intent or underlying purpose.

People need to be able to keep in touch, but having to direct all communication through a social work or adoption agency is not effective. Many services are part-time, social workers take leave, are sick, go on courses or just leave. They are simply not available enough to be an effective channel for communication, hence our particular encouragement of e-mail. We are also convinced that most birth/adoptive family relationships do not need social work support, intervention or management, most of the time. If we can leave those who can to manage their own family business while they are happy to for much of the time, we then have the space to concentrate our time and efforts on the most difficult and complex situations that need most support. The primary aim of having the birth and adoptive families in touch with each other is so they can arrange for themselves what form contact between them shall take. At some times, depending on health, location and other commitments simply exchanging an occasional e-mail will be the only communication. In other situations using e-mail to arrange dates, times, venues and activities for a physical get together of several family members

154

will prove invaluable. Because it is almost instant e-mail is also a useful means of double-checking arrangements at the last minute or letting someone know if something unforeseen has happened that requires the arrangements to be changed or postponed.

We noted that adopters are very concerned that birth relatives may be unreliable and children will be let down and disappointed. Our approach to this is to encourage the family not simply to arrange to meet but to meet to do something together. Going to a pantomime in the Christmas school holidays is a popular activity, new family films tend to be released for the school summer holidays and theme parks, zoos and the like are often less crowded during the Easter holidays than in the summer. This way of working moves the focus from the individuals to the activity. The plan can be to meet outside an attraction, or just inside if there is difficulty over who will be expected to pay. If after a pre-agreed waiting time the people expected do not arrive the activity goes ahead as planned anyway and the day is not lost. Sure the children involved will have learned something about people's unreliability but that is a reality they need to be aware of – at least they cannot blame Mum for not trying. Receipt of an e-mail when they return home explaining what prevented the rendezvous will help ameliorate negative feelings before they become entrenched.

We are firmly convinced that venues that have no institutional overtone are best. Who really wants to return to a family centre that has unhappy memories or to have to perch on tiny playgroup chairs? Places where children can run and shout or laugh loudly are great because they allow tension to be released in a physical way. We also recommend a fairly tight time scale as no one can know in advance how an event will work out. Advance planning just to see the film can always be extended to going for tea or onto a park if everyone is comfortable and wants to stay together longer but no one is offended if the original plan has to be followed because of prior commitments.

One family we worked with meets at a family diner pub with a big play barn and outdoor area. The arrangement was for the adoptive mother and two adopted daughters of about 10 and 12 to meet up with birth mother, big brother who was about 16 and little half-brother who was 4, at midday for lunch. The 4-year-old heads for the play barn and the 10-year-old quickly follows. The two older children try to look sophisticated with their cokes but quickly bore and resolve the situation by offering to 'take the little ones' onto the adventure playground equipment and look after them until the meals are ready. Left alone the two women update each other on wider family events and progress at school. As frequently happens, the birth mother needs some help with a form from the Benefits Agency. Some people may question the appropriateness of the adoptive mother being caught up in this but a more positive interpretation is that she is both willing and able to help. Her daughters like to see that their adoptive mother is helpful to their birth mother and it creates a climate of warmth and respect in which all can flourish. This particular birth mother had recurrent mental health problems.

If she was very depressed she may say quite worrying things and ask inappropriate questions. However, when in the pub she actually spent very little time in direct conversation with the girls; the person bearing the brunt of any unhappiness is the adoptive mother who once said 'Her shoulders were broad enough to take it'. So if the birth mother was low, after more play for the kids while the women have a coffee, the 'two hours three times a year contact' is fulfilled. If she is well, lively and energetic, the adoptive mum will suggest a walk across the fields to a local country park and the meeting extends to a full half day that is enjoyed by everyone. This is a good example of what can be achieved with goodwill and flexibility. It also illustrates that someone needs to be acknowledged to be the organiser, not in charge and carrying all responsibility but still to be the recognised leader.

We have also found that not all the family members need to do everything together. One grandmother who is caring for her eldest grandson was described in very negative terms by a local authority. Her two younger grandchildren were to be adopted and while the grandmother supported the plan she was unhappy about the local authority's implementation. We were asked to mediate. We were warned that under no circumstances should she learn the identity or address of the adopters. They met. Grandma liked the adopters. The adopters liked and respected her for her advocacy on behalf of the children. The one obvious thing they had in common was a shared lack of regard for social workers which we worked hard to overcome. Two years on and we are no longer involved. They meet frequently and the adoptive father takes his son and the elder brother to a first division football match. Grandma, adoptive mother and the youngest child, a little girl who hates football, go shopping for fun and pretty things. So positive is the relationship that the Grandma has named the adopters as guardians of the eldest boy and he has the security of knowing that if his beloved Grandma is ever unable to carry on caring for him he will have a home with his brother and sister.

So what does the West Midlands Post-Adoption Service consider the essential elements of contact arrangements in the twenty-first century?

- A shared commitment to keep in touch.
- A positive commitment not to lose touch.
- Easy access to support, assistance, guidance and mediation if and when needed.
- The freedom to manage the situation independent of third parties if preferred.
- Choice of means of communication.
- One person willing to act as organiser.
- Adults being willing to be flexible and prepared to make adjustments to benefit all the children involved.
- Financial support to ensure everyone can afford 'events'.
- Recognition that just being together can be 'a good thing'.

- Recognition that the various people involved will bring different things on different occasions and each will take different things away.
- A belief that being in touch is preferable to not being in touch in the long term and being willing to overcome irritations and hiccups to achieve this.
- An attitude of openness and sense of connection shared by all involved.

Sadly, we know we have an uphill struggle to achieve this as we only encounter people after adoption – the work to ensure the right attitudes needs to happen much earlier. There are two opportunities that must not be missed.

Openness of heart and mind must be inherent in the recruitment and preparation of adopters and within the attitudes of staff involved. People should not be asked 'how much contact can you accept?' They should learn how birth families are important to children, a birth family may be abusing, it may be neglectful but it is theirs and that is important. They should learn from their earliest encounter with adoption agencies that we now know that it is important for children and adults who are adopted to be able to keep in touch with birth families wherever possible. They should be asked not if but how they would envisage keeping in touch with birth families. We should change the emphasis from suggesting no contact is the easy option to making it clear that lack of contact is a problem area. Ask anyone who has adopted, or was, an 'abandoned baby'. They will know the real cost of being devoid of contact or information. We should ask the question: 'Would you be able to parent a child who cannot or does not have continuing communication with birth family members and face all the potential problems this lack of information and sense of identity may bring?'. While professionals continue to see contact as inherently problematic we will never recruit the pool of adopters who, presented with a different scenario from the outset, would transfer learning from family situations in general and be positive about keeping in touch.

It would be no use having adopters welcoming steps to keep in touch if many birth parents are lost before a child's adopters are identified. We must hold on to birth parents through the adoption process by providing an independent worker to support them and if necessary advocate on their behalf. We must make a distinction between the adversarial court-based processes leading to care and adoption orders from the adoption preparation essential for all the birth relatives who will have continuing connections with the child. This work must also be undertaken when a child or baby is being relinquished for adoption. We must make sure that no one forgets that creating another human being also creates a connection and a degree of responsibility that can never be wiped out by any court order.

References

Howe, D. and Feast, J. (2000), *Adoption, search and reunion: the long-term experience of adopted adults*, London, Children's Society.

19

WITH LOVE

Jane French

I married a man who was adopted. I chose him over my long term boyfriend because I thought he needed me more. He managed to bypass the normal process of getting to know each other while 'going out' and somehow just moved in on my life. Briefly a part of my mind knew that he was behaving like deprived children I had met in my work, offering affection to strangers freely – which even though it was endearing, was inappropriate. But I wasn't listening to reason and his overwhelming 'thereness' must have engaged with some emotional need in me. We talked a lot in those early days about how we would bring up children. We cared very much about how it should be, he shared his books on child psychology with me. We both wanted to parent better than the way we had experienced it ourselves. His unhappy experience was obvious and mine had been far too cold and English middle class, being looked after by successive nannies and au pairs. I remember looking up and saying 'Mummy, mummy' in a pleading sort of way and the nanny saying to my mother 'Leave her, it's just power they want'. We were determined that our children would have that power to demand and expect love.

We ended up living together after only a few weeks and married a year later. I wore my granny's Victorian petticoat as a dress and I dressed him in a Welsh miner's shirt. He didn't really want relatives there as he didn't want the contrast between mine and his, but relented at the last minute for parents and siblings only. We had a happy wedding and I made all the food in heart shapes, it was colourful and filled with children and friends – the sort of wedding people who live together have when they're not sure if they believe in marriage or not. Three weeks after our wedding when I was deliriously happy and in love he had his first affair and while I was having our second child he had another, and there were more. Other people thought we must have been unhappy together for it to happen, but it was often when we were particularly happy and getting on well.

Glad to have left the dating game far behind, I was very content with a lovely husband and two gorgeous children but he still seemed to have needs I did not have. I felt that he was continually searching for something, an emotional completeness much as a rooting baby searches for the breast. That feeling of being at one with the world and total contentment had never been his and instinctively he rooted for it for many years. I suspect that no-one would ever have been the 'right' partner for him for long because it was really the right mothering experience he needed which would have made the world seem right for him. It was the warmth and smell and closeness of an infant with its mother and the total understanding and close communication with a parent which he had always lacked. That hole in him could never be filled more than temporarily.

Childbirth was always a dangerous time in our relationship. It seemed to throw up very strong and angry feelings in him, far removed from the blissful happiness of other couples at that time. He was, of course, delighted when his first real blood relative was born. But on the day I came home with our baby he chose to confess to his affair of four years ago, when we had first been married. With our second child, I was horrified later to discover that at my check-up when she was six weeks old, I had to be treated for a sexually transmitted infection. The whole mother–baby scenario was problematic for him in some way. I think it reminded him of what he had never had, the deep hurt, the pain of separation and never becoming really connected with his adoptive mother.

I know that many people are happily and successfully adopted by special, caring parents who are loving and empathetic people, because I know some like that. However, my husband's adoptive parents were wrong for him. The difference in their intelligence was extreme, and brown hair was their only matching feature. When I met them I was surprised they expressed their disappointment at not being able to have children 'of their own' and adoption was obviously a 'second best'. I thought they should have been delighted and have known how lucky they were to have such a gorgeous, intelligent and good-looking son, the man I was in love with.

They seemed to like the trappings of parenthood best, the pram, the DIY, behaving like the neighbours. They told a story where they went to the shops together and bought two doughnuts for themselves. On the way back, my husband started eating one of them. 'How sweet, you didn't realise he was old enough to want one', I thought. 'Did you go back and get another?' No, the whole point of the story was that he was very naughty to have taken theirs. I had toddlers at the time and thought how strange it was not to laugh and enjoy him doing that. They were never the kind of parents who said 'Don't come over today, the roads are icy and dangerous', they wanted us to go anyway as the son next door had visited twice that week. When one of our children was a baby she covered her nose and mouth with her hand when someone she did not know went very close to her. She did not seem to like the smell of them. His adoptive mother said he used to do that all the time when she went near him and she had decided that it was because he felt 'ashamed of being a bastard'. I found that a very shocking idea and wondered if they conveyed that to him during his childhood.

Communications between them never seemed to progress beyond a very basic level. He seemed to lack any real contact with them, there being nothing in common and no similarities. He never learned to talk, argue and discuss in his family as a means of negotiation or of sharing. His parents were locked into their domestic routines, which made their lives appear normal. He once told me of a time he had been travelling round Europe in the holidays and having had all his money stolen he had to hitch hike home from Italy, starving and penniless. On arriving exhaustedly at the door, his mother said: 'Aren't you lucky, it's a quarter to nine and we have cocoa at nine'. What mother would not have delightedly made a meal for her son at any time of the day or night? From what he has told me, he learned to live with himself. In his bedroom he read literature, poetry, politics and philosophy. He listened to the World Service and all kinds of music. He educated himself and against all the odds, he won an Open Scholarship to Oxford. I later read some letters he wrote to his parents from there. They were intelligent, informative and sensitive letters, as if he was still seeking their affection and approval. One bit in them really saddened me; in it he pleads with his parents to come and collect him on a certain day before the May Ball because he doesn't want to be there as he can't afford to go. What parent would not have been so proud to have their son at Oxford that they would not have found the money somehow? They weren't having to support him, he had a grant, and he worked to earn money in the holidays.

The relationship engaged feelings of guilt and obligation more than real empathy and communication. We always had to see them much more than my family or our friends and it was often a bit joyless and laden with reproach. However long we stayed it was never long enough. Nothing ever filled the real emptiness for them or for him. They were never the right parents for him. Looking back I don't think they could really cope with such an intelligent teenager. He used words they didn't understand, they couldn't readily engage with him either, and it made them more helpless in relation to him. Their need to be parents seemed more important than the needs of their child.

His birth mother had tried to keep in touch at first but they had asked the adoption society to tell her not to write any more – they wanted no contact. Many years later he did find his birth mother and some half siblings, which was a great success. She looked the same, was a very warm person and we were very welcomed; they were all obviously 'family'. But it was too late for deep emotional needs to be fulfilled – they couldn't regress to his babyhood and start again. They had both missed out. Something I noticed about his birth mother was that she was much more skilled in subtly modifying the behaviour of her children and having expectations. She asked people to move up at the table, make room for each other, to share. She played a more educative and socialising role.

We have been together for twenty-six years now and I was beginning to think that he could be happy with me but sadly I know now that he is still searching. Perhaps I can never fill the deep hurt inside him and the hurt will be passed on, not just to me but also to our two children. I think he lives with us but mostly with himself – he is very successful in his work and he has interests he enjoys which take up all his time. He is a workaholic and he is brilliant in a great many different and difficult aspects of his career. I think enormous success and achievement have saved him from feeling the powerless abandoned baby he once was. I am really proud of him.

Like in his adoptive family, I suspect, he is a bit apart from us and doubts my relevance to his life. I was looking forward to our time alone together after our children have grown up, when I could stop being so much of a mother and be able to care more for him, go out together, enjoy ourselves as adults. Our children are on the cusp of their adult lives, optimistic, bright, confident and beautiful and I know they will be so hurt by what he is planning to do. We've brought them up together and he should feel so proud. Fathers give daughters confidence and have the power to take it away too. We're nearly there and he's off again.

He wants to start again, a new life. Unfortunately, I still love him and I want to make him happy, somehow. He says he doesn't love me any more, but he was never one for saying he loved me, anyway. Quite early on in our marriage he said, a bit like Prince Charles to Diana, that he didn't know what love felt like. I think it feels like him making me a cup of coffee in the morning or giving me something I would like to read. I think that is love and I would like to love him back if he would let me. Because he has hurt my feelings on occasions, I have been less able to show it than I would like. But on one level I do understand that as the mother he most wanted as a baby wasn't loyal to him, why should he be loyal to me?

Part IV

THE POLITICS OF ADOPTION

INTRODUCTION

A statement by the Prime Minister about adoption is now as likely to get as much media attention as one on law and order or taxation. At first sight, this is curious. After all, the number of children available for adoption is comparatively small. These children constitute a tiny fraction of the total numbers of children in care and parliamentarians hardly get exercised about the majority of those children. Indeed, given that more than half of them are in foster care, where is the debate about that? In the year ending March 2000, 3,135 children were adopted in England, which showed a steady increase from 1999 (2,880) and 1999 (2,410) (*Hansard*, 2001). At most, 5,000 children can be adopted out of a projected nearly 60,000 children in the care system over the next 5–10 years. The more noise about adoption, the quieter the voices of the other 55,000 children.

Every child is entitled to protection, well being and a loving family but the numbers of children needing adoption produce a disproportionate response. It also seems unlikely that even the practised oratory of Paul Boateng who, when Health Minister, was adoption's stoutest parliamentary champion, could bring the citizenry to the barricades with his condemnation of all the politically correct ills that social work is allegedly heir to when it deals with would-be adoptive parents.

That adoption is a matter of enormous public, media and political interest there can be no doubt. That it is generally regarded as a Good Thing is also beyond dispute. Well, almost. It is curious that Patricia Morgan, one of the fiercest opponents of what she alleges are the shortcomings of social work and local authority adoption practice could write as late as 1998: 'Adoption has fallen out of favour ... It is under attack as a childcare strategy by a powerful alliance of feminists, child care professionals, racial awareness campaigners and the media' (Morgan, 1998). Ms Morgan has rounded up the usual suspects to make the case against liberalism but any reading of newspapers further back than 1998 would indicate that the media would have a good case to seek a magistrate's ruling that they be released from this band.

165

There are, of course, those aspects of the unconscious, myth and the psyche which generate an understandably human interest in adoption and we have referred to these in the introduction to this book. Adoption is also a matter of human interest. For some years inter-country adoption, until very recently a fairly unregulated practice, provided the occasional human interest. And then there are those occasional dramas which are served up to television viewers and newspaper readers with the regularity of a TV soap opera. In 1999, the Bramleys went on the run with two children whom Cambridgeshire social services department were refusing to allow them to adopt. In 2001, there were the protracted goings-on of the Kilshaws with their so-called 'Internet twins'. This threw in car journeys across the American badlands, characters who might have inhabited a Denis Hopper film, an embarrassing but enlightening piece of television verité, and the Kilshaws' eventual bankruptcy for good measure.

But this is part of the day-to-day diet of newspaper coverage – if adoption does not offer the human interest, something else will. For some time, too, occasional media stories have been run about the alleged political correctness of social workers who supposedly refuse to approve as adoptive parents overweight people, those who were too middle class, the wrong race, who smoked or even those who had too many books in their homes. But what is interesting about adoption, given that it fuels the political correctness debate (if such a word can be used to dignify what is largely media mud-slinging and political mischief-making) is that adoption has not always been the vehicle for attacks on social work and political correctness is a fairly recent hammer with which to beat social work.

In 1991, Franklin and Parton (1991) published *Social Work, The Media and Public Relations*. There were, unsurprisingly, many accusations against social workers which they and their fellow contributors were able to excavate through very careful research but the charge of political correctness was not one of them. The same occurred when Franklin revisited the territory (Franklin, 1998). Looking at newspaper coverage of social work and social services he found that reporting was overwhelmingly negative and reported instances of negative words and phrases, some of them occurring hundreds of times in the newspapers, quality and tabloid, which he surveyed. These included 'abusing trust', 'negative', 'incompetent', 'negligent', 'failed', 'ineffective', 'misguided', 'bungling', 'naïve', 'left wing'. However, 'politically correct' did not occur often enough (though it did occur) to appear in his tables. The reason for this could be that the period of his survey did not feature any controversy (for example, about adoption) where critics thought it the appropriate phrase of opprobrium.

What one can read from the work of Franklin and Parton, who have done much of the research on the media and social work, is that child protection is the main source of media criticism of social work (the afore-quoted negative words and phrases were almost wholly applied to that area), and that political correctness is almost wholly applied to adoption. (In the distant past, though political correctness was not then the word in vogue, local authorities, attitudes to, and policies on race were vehicles for criticism.)

But whatever actual faults social workers and local authorities might be guilty of, when it comes to criticising them over adoption, some critics are not deterred from dragging up an infamous case even when it is known there was found to be no case to answer – the case of Jim and Roma Lawrence. Two prominent critics of social work – one from the inside and one from the outside – have done this in recent times. Melanie Phillips, the *Daily Mail* columnist, tends to regard social work as either one of the ills of modern society and/or one of its causes. Professor Robert Pinker of the London School of Economics has a distinguished career as a social work teacher (although he is not, interestingly, a qualified social worker). He has been a fierce critic of what he has seen as the excesses of social work as exhibited in the now defunct Central Council for Education and Training in Social Work. He has also criticised the grandiose ambitions of social work, against the more modest, casework model which he has advocated (Pinker, 1982). He is also the privacy commissioner and a member of the Press Complaints Commission. For Phillips and Parker, the Lawrences were a godsend.

Jim Lawrence is a white Englishman and Roma, his wife, was born in Guyana. In 1993 they were living in Cromer in Norfolk and wanted to adopt a mixed-race child. They claimed they were turned down as prospective adopters because Mrs Lawrence told their social worker that she had not experienced racism in their home town of Cromer in Norfolk. The adoption panel subsequently advised them that they were 'too racially naïve' to be trusted to bring up a child who was not their own (Pinker, 1993).

In response to outrage in the media, the then Health Secretary, Virginia Bottomley ordered an investigation. In September 1993 it was officially concluded that the Norfolk adoption panel had given 'due and careful consideration' to the Lawrence's application and that they had been turned down because of the need to keep 'the interest and welfare of the children paramount' – a legal duty placed upon local authorities by the Children Act, 1989, which was passed by a Conservative government.

Despite this official exoneration, both Pinker (Pinker, 1993, 1999) and Phillips (Phillips, 1994) cited the case of Jim and Roma Lawrence as evidence of the malaise which affects and infects social work. In her contribution to a book on political correctness, Melanie Phillips supported her case against the 'illiberal liberals' who, according to her infrared camera, inhabit the public (especially social) services, by using the case of the Lawrences as an illustration. She went on to say that Mrs Lawrence's statement that she had never experienced racism showed 'the surreal world of political correctness [whereby] it is, of course, impossible for a black person not to encounter racism. So that person's experiences must be denied.'

However, worse than this disregard for the facts, came in 1996; worse because the Lawrence case started to be recycled to a wider audience than those who read quasi-academic books and also because politicians now began to use the case illustratively. Indeed, this latter fact marked the beginnings of adoption moving from media interest to being cited by politicians as an ideological tool of social work. That year the Junior Health Minister, John Bowis announced that 'political correctness has no place in the adoption process' and announced an Adoption Bill, which, in the event, never reached the statute book. *The Times* covered the story by a case study of the Lawrences, which was headed 'Pair defeated by "political correctness"' (*The Times*, 29 March 1996).

The amnesia affecting the media and others seemed to be infectious because in 1997 it inflicted Stephen Dorrell, Mrs Bottomley's successor at the Health Department, when he unveiled a White Paper (Department of Health, 1997) when a general election was expected to be called at any time. The *Daily Mail* wrote of 'sweeping changes aimed at driving political correctness out of the adoption process will be announced by Stephen Dorrell today' (*Daily Mail*, 17 February 1997). And, perhaps to no one's surprise, out from the files came a photograph of the Lawrences under the headline: 'Couple punished for success'. This suggested that their middle class status and material comfort had been held against them, as well as Mrs Lawrence's statement about her experience of a lack of racial prejudice. Mr Dorrell was not to be outdone by the tabloids. He, too, used the case in radio interviews when defending his new policies. Alas, he never thought to consult his departmental records or, if he did, he chose to ignore them.

The Lawrence case is not only interesting for its bar room-handiness when it comes to arguments about adoption. It raises two other issues. Citing a (in this case) false case over and over again can give the impression that there is more than one instance of the flaw one is attempting to correct.

But such a case also illustrates the problems a local authority can face when it turns people down. The Lawrences' complaints were the subject of an official inquiry. Others which surface are not and come and go with the next day's edition. In the generality of cases, the aggrieved couple state their side of the story. There may be reasons for rejection which might seem valid which the public would at first sight query. Is smoking a good enough reason? Well, it might be if it were excessive and injurious to the parents' (even the child's) health. People over the age of 40 can and do adopt but is it wise to encourage too many people to be dealing with teenage children when they are in their sixties and seventies? These are reasonable arguments. Some applicants, though, when turned down do not take it lightly. Who would? Who would wish to be told by a committee that you are judged inadequate to care for a child? That they go to the newspapers is understandable. That they tell the newspapers only part of the story, that they place interpretations on reasons is also understandable. But what is a local authority to do – betray the confidentiality of those discussions and wash the couples' dirty linen in public? To place the public standing of the organisation against the short-comings of individuals who have to continue to see their neighbours every day, people whom the authority will know are not malicious but distressed and disappointed?

But for all that adoption remains vastly misunderstood at the same time that its face has so greatly changed. The issues which surround modern adoption, the philosophies which underlie it, the kind of practice demanded of the modern social worker, even the kinds of children now available for adoption – all of these are still largely hidden from the public and ignored by the media. And yet given the comparatively small number of children involved, adoption merits swathes of newsprint and hours of parliamentary time.

There are, of course, reasonable critisms to be made of practice, policy and law, some of which will be resolved by the Adoption and Children Act. But much remains to be done. For example, in this part, a contributor challenges the concept of permanence, seeing it as a product of politics and culture. Mary Austin, who adopted two children, one from overseas and one with special needs from within the UK, talks about how attachments develop between adopters and the children who come to live with them. Her daughter, Julia, describes how being transracially adopted feels to a young person in the UK today. Angela Howard and Sheena and Donald Macrae describe the frustrations and joys of adopting from overseas. Chris Hanvey questions the value of adoption panels. Finally, Anna Gupta reviews progress for black and ethnic minority children in the UK child care system, and concludes that whilst progress has been made, much more needs to be done.

In 1996, as previously mentioned, the Conservative government published abortive proposals to review adoption law. However, the present government's commitment saw a review chaired by no less a figure than the Prime Minister himself. This was rapidly followed by the Adoption and Children Act, which fell with the dissolution of parliament in May 2001. But the wish to give a legislative prod to local authorities is such that the Bill was among the first to be reintroduced of that year and passed into law in 2002.

Much of the pressure for change has come from a group of (mainly) Conservative MPs, notable among whom is Julian Brazier. This may account for the fact that while social work has, more or less embraced the latest reforms, it cannot have been said to have been in the forefront of those calling for them. The profession also retreated into a corner in the face of the onslaught of no-nonsense criticism levelled at it by Paul Boateng, when Junior Health Minister. For him, social workers were the politically correct frustrators of common sense adoption policies. The key to adoption, he said, was the ability of would-be adoptive parents to 'love and care' whatever their weight, personal habits, class or (importantly) race (Boateng, 1998). He went on:

> Local authorities still refuse to place children for adoption because
> one of the prospective partners is 40-plus, or smokes, or is deemed
> too middle class, the wrong colour, or the expectation of the child
> is too high. All of these so-called reasons are in themselves nothing
> more than excuses. A couple should only be turned down if there
> are sound and defensible reasons for doing so.
>
> (Boateng, 1998)

In fact, though Paul Boateng promised that new adoption guidelines would stop all this politically correct nonsense, they were far more temperate than his language. The National Adoption Standards (Department of Health, 2001) issued in 2001 say no more than that applicants must be treated 'without prejudice' and 'fairly, openly and with respect'. It adds that no one should be excluded on any ground other than criminal. That is as wide or as narrow as you care to define it. The Bill leaves matters where they are. While there were things which Boateng stated with which most people, not least social workers, would agree, even if he presented them as matters of controversy, there was no evidence that hard and fast rules were being applied. Thus, cool analysis of what actually does happen has won out over political rhetoric.

Some couples also complain of the 'bureaucracy' they have to face at the hands of local authorities, another charge eagerly taken up by critics and called 'red tape' in the tabloids. But this frequently overlooks the fact that adoption is a service for children and is not to satisfy the needs of those who are childless or who, having children of their own, wish to adopt.

It is a curiosity in this field that few, if any of the criticisms about political correctness, bureaucracy and the other sins which local authorities are said to be heir to, are made of voluntary adoption agencies, significant among whom are the Catholic diocesan agencies. Yet these agencies are bound by the same laws and procedures as govern local authorities, and their workers will most probably have worked for a local authority and will certainly have studied on the same social work qualification courses as their local authority colleagues. Voluntary adoption agencies are the respectable face of adoption practice. In the political mind, local authorities are disrespectability personified.

There are many reasons why adoption commands political and public attention, not least because a life in our public care system rarely benefits the children who endure it, and adoption appears to, and can, offer a better life. On the other hand, as we have stated, there are more than 58,000 children and young people who are looked after by local authorities but not only will the overwhelming majority not be adopted – they are not available for adoption. As we have said in our introduction, adoption also strikes those chords of identity, place, selfhood and myth which are important to us as human beings, which influence us and shape our lives. As an anvil on which to beat social work, adoption has proven a trusty instrument. Most people will tend to side with the couple spurned by the allegedly insensitive and politically correct bureaucracy when the 'facts' are presented, as they usually are, simplistically. In this field there are none of the ambiguities which afflict the media and political concern with child protection; the dilemma of being damned if they do act, and damned if they don't. No, adoption offers vulnerable children in need loving and altruistic parents. And while there must be cases of social workers making decisions for the wrong reasons – how could there not be? – these are not the standard fare of social work practice. Yet such instances – and more the myths, distortions and falsehoods – condemn a whole profession in a way that even Harold Shipman has not turned the local GP into a feared ogre or Robert Maxwell has not created the myth of the crooked business-man. No, adoption, used in this way, is a mere convenience, a weapon to hand. If it were not adoption, it would be something else.

But, as in the case of child protection, the constant dripping of criticism weareth away a profession. Social workers, we know, become defensive and reactive in their practice. There is now plenty of reasons to believe that constant media criticism, which finds its echoes in the House of Commons, has a deleterious effect on the recruitment of social workers, contributing to what is now a crisis. And if it does social workers no good, whatever does it do for the long-term interests of those whom society employs them to serve – the child in care, the birth parent and the prospective adopter?

References

Boateng, P. (1998), Adoption is never black and white, *Daily Express*, 12 April.

Department of Health (1997), *Achievement and challenge*, London, The Stationery Office.

Department of Health (2001), *National adoption standards*, London, The Stationery Office.

Franklin, B. (1998), *Hard pressed: national newspaper reporting of social work and Social Services*, Sutton, *Community Care*/Reed Business Publishing.

Franklin, B. and Parton, N. (eds) (1991), *Social work, the media and public relations*, London, Routledge.

Hansard (2001), 6 November, Col. 235W.

Morgan, P. (1998), *Adoption and the care of children: the British and American expe-rience*, London, Institute for Economic Affairs.

Phillips, M. (1994), Illiberal liberalism, in Dunant, S. (ed.) *The war of words*, London, Virago.

Pinker, R. (1982), An alternative view, in Barclay, P. (ed.) *Social work: its roles and tasks*, London, Bedford Square Press/National Institute for Social Work.

Pinker, R. (1993), A lethal kind of looniness, *Times Higher Education Supplement*, 10 September.

Pinker, R. (1999), Social work and adoption: a case of mistaken identities, in Philpot, T. (ed.), *Political correctness and social work*, London, IEA Health and Welfare Unit.

20

THE FICTION OF PERMANENCE

Adele Jones

The concept of permanence first took root in the US in the 1970s (Barry and Pelton, 1994) and soon became an important principle of child welfare practice both within the UK (Thoburn, 1980) as well as in other countries. The concept is based on the view that children benefit from living in stable, loving family environments that can last indefinitely. While it is expected that as children mature the role of family and their role within family will alter, it is nevertheless assumed that the importance of family has life-long significance for most people and provides the best opportunities for meeting the needs of children.

Permanence has been defined as:

> the systematic process of carrying out, within a brief, time-limited period, a set of goal-directed activities designed to help children live in families that offer continuity of relationships with nurturing parents or caretakers and the opportunity to establish life-time relationships.
>
> (Maluccio *et al.*, 1986)

When birth families are unable to provide the type of environment or stability required it is generally accepted that alternative forms of care should seek as far as possible to emulate the sense of permanence that upbringing in a family can bring. Research findings highlighting the perceived successes of the lives of adopted children has led in the UK to permanence being increasingly linked to adoption (Department of Health, 1993). Studies which point to factors such as higher educational achievement and lower levels of crime among adopted children compared to children in local authority care tend to minimise the fact that adoption usually means an improvement in opportunity and economic status and it is these factors as much as the family context which accounts for this. These links between social deprivation and other social problems are so well established they do not need restating.

Nevertheless, social policy within the UK now dictates that consideration is given to permanence through adoption as an option for children who cannot receive a satisfactory standard of care within their birth families. The rationale for this development is presented as being so 'sound', it is assumed that there is little need for debate.

Permanence is presented as a concept about which there is universal consensus, universal application and as if it was a measurable fixed entity. The concept is not unproblematic however and despite its apolitical and neutral pretensions, the lack of discussion about the contradictions and dilemmas it contains may be one of the factors behind the steady increase in the number of adoptions in which parental consent is dispensed with (Fratter, 1996). Furthermore, underscrutinised claims have made it possible for the concept to be appropriated by politicians and policy makers so that in government policy, we see permanence reduced to its most functional aspects, as in the introduction of the market concepts of objectives and targets in increasing adoption placements for children. While there may be benefits of such a focus in terms of greater attention to planning and resources, adoption, particularly in the circumstances outlined above 'represents the most forceful of interventions by the state into family life' (Charlton *et al.*, 1998, p. 3). For this reason alone if for no other, it is important to dislodge and question the 'certainties' that are the basis of current policy.

Permanence, is not so much 'common sense' knowledge, as a social work construct that was developed out of concerns about the 'drift' associated with children cared for in children's homes and foster homes and negative outcomes in terms of lack of stability, changes of placement, loss of contact with birth family and other problems such as poor educational attainment and behavioural and emotional difficulties (Barry and Pelton, 1994). The concept is now so strongly embedded within social work practice that the phrase 'permanency movement' is commonly stated within social work literature (Barry and Pelton, 1994). This is an indication of the groundswell of support among practitioners who promote permanence as natural and beneficial to children. The benefits of permanence, however, cannot be explained as if the facts speak for themselves.

Adoption has the effect of removing the birth parent's rights, responsibilities and legal connections to a child and at the same time conferring these upon the adoptive parents. Because this process is irreversible and immutable it satisfies at one level, that of policy objective, the commitment to providing a permanent home for children. This presupposes that by permanence one is simply referring to a legal fact, establishing a child's legal status and position within a family he or she was not born in to. If however, permanence refers to the attachment, sense of belonging and stability that being part of a family can bring, then the focus on adoption in achieving this is too limiting. Within many societies, belonging and identity are not concepts that are easily removed from the context of the birth family, so that a child may remain permanently connected as a member of their birth family although their permanent home may be with another family. Permanence carries different meanings depending upon the social and cultural contexts within which they arise. The construct in social work terms makes use of a conflation of different factors that are not necessarily mutually exclusive, but neither are they mutually dependent. These factors can be described as: material concerns, that is where and with whom a child lives, the child's physical and emotional care; discourses about belonging, identity and ideologies of family. That the term carries several meanings simultaneously or interchangeably is less important than the ways in which specific meanings are emphasised or minimised for particular ends. So, birth parents may be forced to relinquish their children if they are unable to guarantee permanency in terms of the material conditions and care provided; yet permanency in terms of a sense of belonging may be sustained. Placement with adoptive parents on the other hand, carries the expectation of permanency, yet there are no penalties should they not succeed. The relinquishing of children in these circumstances is less likely to be as a consequence of state intervention. The only certainty is that adoptive families fit perceptions of the type of family able to provide permanency!

'Permanence' then does not have a fixed meaning about which there is agreement; and indeed its significance in social work terms has grown over time. Its value and meaning depends upon the cultural, social and historical context in which it is situated. This raises questions about the ways in which literature on the subject promotes experience and studies based on ethnocentric perceptions and assumptions as universal 'knowledge' about what is best for children.

Families are themselves impermanent. It is not simply that they are constantly changing, it is that the provision of a stable family life, the aim of the permanency movement, is something that many families are unable to sustain. Although there are no studies to draw on, experiential evidence suggests, for example, that when relationships between adoptive parents break down, it is unlikely that the commitment to the child, assured at the time of the adoption, or even contact, will be sustained equally by both parties. It is also the case that marital problems between adoptive parents are a factor in the breakdown of some adoptive placements (Livingston Smith and Howard, 1999). After the death of adoptive parents, their children may not be able to take it for granted that they have a permanent place in the extended family. This is because the making of a statutory adoption order may achieve the objectives for permanence set by social workers and policy makers but it does not create or affirm permanence for families either in terms of lived reality or lifelong attachment within a family network. The relationships within and between families are mediated through, and affected by a host of other factors and are specific to families rather than to policy.

Some adoptive parents and adopted children carry with varying levels of intensity and for many years, the feeling that 'this is not going to last', or that they wish to end it at some point. Adoptive families are especially vulnerable to disruption particularly when the behaviour of the child tests the limits of the family's emotional resources and relationships (Livingston Smith and Howard, 1999). It is the fear of impermanence rather than a belief in permanence that usually hangs like a cloud at these times, sometimes for years. When children are determined to see what it takes for them to be rejected, adoptive parents and social workers offer the reassurance that 'this is your forever family'; this is where the cycle of destruction, rejection and removal ends. I suspect this is more for the benefit of the adults than for the child, since the child knows with more certainty than anyone that breakdown is possible. There was a time when the child and the adoptive parents existed without each other, the child is aware that returning to local authority care is not an irrational fear, it happens, and while reassurance is a necessary bridge for holding on, it is not the 'truth', for this cannot be known. The salve is temporary, it is usually only a deeper healing that can make permanence become 'more true'. Also, children may have strong mutually loving relationships with their adoptive family yet at the same time, retain the feeling of being permanently connected to their birth family. It is not in the designs of children to go along with adults who would seek to create permanent families through adoption as if the child had no connection to any other family. If we were to consider permanence in the context of birth families, we would find that as an abstract notion, it is the child, rather than the adult who owns the idea of permanence whereas in adoptive families, the notion is conferred and is not always owned by the child.

Where the notion of permanence has value to children and families, it is as an expression of the connectedness a child and family may feel to one another, the commitment and strength of relationships that exist and an acceptance that this is one's place. It is important to acknowledge the complexity of what is happening here. This form of permanence is not the result of a policy objective, it is because an individual child feels connected emotionally to their adoptive family. They have adopted the family as clearly as the parents have adopted them and for the child the concept may be retained at an emotional level even if family life is disrupted. This is significant for three reasons. First, when an adoptive family breaks down there is little support for the parents to sustain emotional connections even though this may be immensely important to the child. Second, such is the pressure on adoptive families to succeed, that parents sometimes demonise the behaviour of their child in order to reduce feelings of guilt and failure and as moral justification to others for 'giving up' (Livingston Smith and Howard, 1999). This makes it very difficult to repair and sustain relationships where this may benefit the child. The consequences in terms of loss, rejection and labelling are damaging for the child and for the parents too whose grieving for the loss of their child may be inhibited or else conducted through a distorted lens. Third, it undermines the rights of the child to family life, for surely they continue to have a right to a family in which they have been permanently placed?

One of the reasons that children's rights in this regard are neglected is because adults involved in adoption processes have negated the importance of their role and contribution to the success of adoption. While consulting with children about their views on adoption is enshrined in practice and policy, the child's role in adoption is generally considered by adults as one that is passive. When children begin to act out their distress with the circumstances of their lives and some of the experiences they have faced however, they are anything but passive. It is at this point that they are likely to become the direct focus of counselling, therapy and other forms of intervention (Livingston Smith and Howard, 1999). The stability that we, as adults, strive for is not achieved by minimising the contribution that children make. They need to be considered as actors in all aspects of adoption processes, not only to become the focus when things go wrong. Children's experiences, particularly in relation to the histories of some adopted children provides evidence of the dominance of adult actions over which the child is able to exercise little control. In most situations and circumstances, children are relatively powerless, however when a child acts out his or her anger and seeks to disrupt the family life it also values, this may be an expression of the child's feelings of powerlessness, but equally, it may be that the child is making use of whatever power is available to him or her. I am not in any sense suggesting that children are responsible when adoptive families break down, for regardless of how it may appear on the surface, behind the most difficult of behaviour presented by children, at some point in the past will usually be the actions of adults that have led to it. There are of course exceptions to this and also situations in which for whatever reasons, the child simply does not wish to remain with the family. Empowering children who are adopted must include empowering them in ways that might help them to exert some control over their lives in ways that are less destructive to themselves. The capacity of a child to exercise power is dependent upon many factors and while it is mostly limited to the localised contexts in which they live their lives, it should not be under-acknowledged.

Studies and inquiries have clearly and consistently pointed up the lack of planning for children in public care (Department of Health, 1991). There is, however, no empirical evidence that lack of planning has been the cause of the problems that children in public care face and neither have there been any studies which link a reduction of these problems with the permanency movement.

While there can be little doubt that the attention to planning, now a requirement for all children in public care in the UK, has often provided the impetus for social workers to work more actively to safeguard children's welfare, it is not at all clear why 'permanence' should be the goal in planning at all.

Although they do not question the value of the concept of permanence, or indeed its meaning Barry and Pelton (1994) draw on studies of adoption disruption in America to argue that the basic intents and purposes of permanency planning have not been met. There is little hard data in the UK on the impact of permanency planning on the placement outcomes of children, yet it is under the auspices of permanence that targets for increased adoptive placements have been introduced.

One of the most important arguments against this development is that with a focus on permanence, preventative services continue to be neglected. Paradoxically, the lack of preventative services is linked to the increased likelihood of a child being adopted:

> There was consensus . . . about the desperate need for family support. Lack of resources had played a large part in whether children were rehabilitated or adopted, and poverty was a common theme for most families.
>
> (Charlton *et al.*, 1998)

Barry and Pelton's findings concur with this. However, they also describe the ways in which a focus on permanence has influenced the nature of social work intervention. Although referring specifically to America, the comments here may equally apply to the UK:

> Our current system is driven primarily by a mandate to investigate parents to determine whether or not their children should be removed from them. It is within this negative, coercive context that the system attempts to help and to gain the trust and co-operation of parents. The investigative/coercive/child-removal role diminishes, hampers and overwhelms the helping role . . . as huge and increasingly larger portions of their budgets are devoted to investigation . . . with little money left over for preventive and supportive services.
>
> (Barry and Pelton, 1994)

Conclusion

Permanence is a concept that has ambiguous, uncertain meaning. Nevertheless it is promoted as if its meaning is fixed and as if its benefits are proven by empirical research. Neither of these is the case, yet the concept has been adopted as a primary objective in policy on children. This is not to say that the concept has no value. What I have attempted to demonstrate is that as the purpose of intervention, the concept masks contradictions, places pressure on both birth and adoptive families to measure up to its expectations and diverts energy and resources away from preventive and supportive services. If we are serious about tackling the impermanence of children's living conditions however, these are precisely the areas that should be the focus of social work with children and families.

References

Barry, M. and Pelton, L. (1994), Has permanency planning been successful? in E. Gambrill and T. Stein (eds) *Controversial issues in child welfare*, Boston, Mass., Allyn and Bacon, pp. 261–74.

Charlton, L., Crank, M., Kansara, K. and Oliver, C. (1998), *Still screaming: birth parents compulsorily separated from their children*, Manchester, After Adoption.

Department of Health (1991), *Patterns and outcomes in child placement: messages from current research and their implications*, London, HMSO.

Department of Health (1993), *Adoption: the future*, London, HMSO.

Fratter, J. (1996), *Adoption with contact: implications for policy and practice*, London, British Agencies for Adoption and Fostering.

Livingston Smith, S. and Howard, J. (1999), *Promoting successful adoptions: practice with troubled families*, Thousand Oaks, CA, Sage.

Maluccio, A. N., Fein, E. and Olmstead, K. A. (1986), *Permanency planning for children: concepts and methods*, London, Routledge, Kegan and Paul.

Thoburn, J. (1980), What kind of permanence? *Adoption and Fostering*, 9, 4.

21

ADOPTION FROM
THE INSIDE

Mary Austin

Our initial experiences of applying to adopt in the UK were distinctly discouraging. The local authority and several adoption agencies painted a dismal picture of a dire shortage of babies and the overwhelming challenges of children with special needs. No doubt social workers saw us as preoccupied with our unexplained infertility and not ready to adopt. Perhaps a different approach to us as potential adopters could have enabled at least one child to find a family at an earlier stage.

We went to Indonesia as a positive alternative to having children, not reckoning on the impact of living in a far more child-focused society than the UK. Everyday conversations began with the question 'how long have you been married?', followed inevitably by 'how many children?' Babies are carried constantly and fed instantly – their needs seemingly accepted and understood. Despite the delights and distractions of adventurous travel, new friendships and interesting work, we found ourselves contemplating adoption again.

The adoption agency in Jakarta was honest if not optimistic. With a general election pending and possible accusations of baby selling, they were not placing children with expatriate families for the time being. If we found a baby, they would support us through the legal process. Few children are available for adoption as extended families are still the norm. A tour of the orphanage convinced us, if we needed convincing, that even transcultural adoption must be better than institutionalised babyhood with little likelihood of later adoption.

Julia came our way with little warning. On Tuesday evening we returned from a holiday in Hong Kong. On Thursday, we tracked down the friend Mark had met by chance at the airport who knew of a baby, due in July or August, possibly needing adoption. On Friday morning we visited the clinic to make enquiries. Ten minutes later, Julia, barely three days old, was in our arms and two hours later after a hasty trip to buy nappies and bottles, we took her home.

We started adoption proceedings, but Julia developed gastro-enteritis that first weekend so keeping her alive took priority. Our memories of the process are entirely positive. Adoption agency and court officials seemed to share our joy in Julia's survival and our good fortune, and the language used in documents and by the court emphasised the benefits of adoption. We wish now we had met Julia's birth mother or been given a photograph: at the time, our feelings were more ambivalent, and the agency advised against meeting, citing possible pressures on us to make a financial contribution which might jeopardise the adoption. Things moved fast and by October, Julia was ours as far as Indonesian law was concerned.

Going home the following year proved more problematic. Britain did not accept Indonesian adoption law so we found ourselves in a Catch 22 situation with Julia deemed stateless, not entitled to a passport or exit visa from either Indonesia or the UK. Our own permits were due to expire. At the very last minute, Indonesia provided our daughter with a travel permit for one year. On the way home we visited Thailand, Bangladesh, India and Nepal: everywhere people showed a friendly fascination in how our new family came to be.

Back in London, proceedings started over again. Naïvely shocked by what we felt was a hostile reception from a social services team which disapproved of transracial adoption and felt we had bypassed systems meant to protect the child, we found much of the process irksome. Julia had to have a medically unnecessary but painful blood test, resulting in screams whenever we went near the surgery. The family study took many hours we felt could have been better spent with families in need, and the court hearing was delayed by officials with limited experience of international law. After a thankfully uneventful hearing, Julia became legally ours for the second time.

Memories of how we came to be considered as parents for Robbie are hazy. Occasionally we responded to advertisements for mixed race children including one for Robbie, then placed with a foster family, and three of his sisters who were in a children's home. A year or so later we were invited to hear more about them. We could not contemplate taking four children, three older than Julia and all with very special needs, but expressed interest in the youngest ones. Concerned we might rush unknowingly into adopting a child with marked learning difficulties, social workers arranged for us to meet Robbie at his school before proceeding further. From the moment Robbie turned to his potential papa and asked winsomely, 'Make me car', we knew that this one was meant to be.

The preparation period was speedy and thorough, if for us, somewhat unreal, and we felt well supported. The adoption panel was held up by industrial action, and I got promoted, planning to start a new job on 1 January the next year. But in early December, two weeks before his sixth birthday, Robbie moved in.

Many aspects of adoption practice proved helpful. Julia helped make a family book to share with Robbie, and came on initial visits. Robbie's adoption book helped us see the positive aspects of his past. My six months' paid adoption leave allowed us to begin to adjust to our new situation, while an adoption allowance for Robbie meant we could plan ahead for one of us to work part-time.

With hindsight there was too much emphasis on the medical aspects of Robbie's disabilities and too little on the practical and emotional aspects of parenting a damaged child. And we all gave too little thought to the needs of our daughter at such a critical time.

We waited impatiently for the required three months before beginning adoption proceedings. All went smoothly until the Friday before the hearing scheduled for Monday, when the possibility of a contested adoption arose. Hustled through a back door into court, the children whisked away, we found that Robbie's birth mother was attending unexpectedly. That day we faced lengthy interrogations and heard recounted the most distressing aspects of Robbie's earliest years. Neither of us had stood in a witness box before. Later we listened, hidden from view, as lawyers questioned Robbie's mother and at the end of the day, the hearing was adjourned. Whilst we were recalled on the Friday of the same week to hear an adoption order being made, we spent that week worrying about what might be going on behind our backs, in solicitors' huddles. The court process was more intimidating because we didn't fully understand it and hadn't been prepared for it. We felt strongly that there must be a better way.

Bringing up adopted children has been different in three main ways. We have tried to incorporate aspects of the children's past histories into our family life. They, and we, have had to deal with identity and attachment issues arising from being adopted across racial and cultural divides, and in Robbie's case, the additional challenges of learning disability and early emotional damage. Finally, we are adjusting to the prospect of excitingly 'different' futures for our children from those we might have anticipated with children of the home-grown kind.

We meet up with Robbie's five siblings twice a year. The two youngest were adopted together as babies; the three older girls spent six years in a children's home before finding a foster family where two of the three still live. Watching these children recover from difficult pasts, and sharing experiences with the other families has been enormously rewarding, though not without challenge. Early visits made me painfully aware that Robbie has the severest needs. I was angry the children had not been taken into care sooner and that almost three vital years were wasted searching to match a family for them. For Robbie and Julia visits caused tension and jealousy as well as excitement and anticipation. Robbie often needed to insist we were seeing his family while Julia felt her role as an 'everyday' sister was being ignored. We often thought about Julia's half-brother and sister at these times.

Giving Julia a sense of Indonesia has been difficult, and we have not done as well as we might. The albums containing her earliest pictures are treasured and shared, and even now I find it hard to resist telling her adoption story. We see friends from Indonesia from time to time. We owe much to the Indonesian Gamelan Music tutors at the Royal Festival Hall where Julia spent Saturday mornings for eleven years, making music with a group of people for whom her Indonesian origins were not entirely strange and who shared a deep love of Indonesia and its culture.

We took Julia, aged seven, to Indonesia the summer before Robbie arrived. She loved staying with our friends in Sulawesi but told us later that in Jakarta she was terrified we might lose her in the crowd and never find her again. On a more recent visit, the constant stares and questioning about her origins we encountered at cafes and stalls were difficult. Staying in upmarket hotels solved some problems but raised wider issues of inequality of which, of course, Julia's own adoption is a part.

In terms of identity and attachment, having Julia as a baby made some things easier. She says she has always felt ours, and that difficulties with her adoption arise more from racism in the UK, while Robbie still expresses frustration that his family can't be together and sustains strong fantasies about his father and grandfather, and, when angry, about how much better life with his 'real' family would be.

Robbie's experience of separation, and lack of early attachments have a huge impact. He continues to seek affection and approval from adults somewhat indiscriminately and though this can be helpful it has its dangers. Shortly after mastering the journey from school, for example, he arrived home one afternoon with a stranger who had convinced Robbie he needed to use our toilet. He still tests out our commitment with temper tantrums, moodiness and a stubbornness that has us and his teachers totally perplexed at times. As professional educators it has been especially hard to have our own child excluded from school.

At the same time, Robbie seems to value enormously being part of our wider family and is wonderfully patient and caring with his aged grandmother for example, despite the frustrations of family gatherings where people sit round talking for huge chunks of time. He loves having other families stay. Julia, on the other hand, shares the family traits of relishing feisty debate and discussion, matches her cousins academically and brings an extra spark of creativity and glamour into the family scene.

We have had to adjust to having a child with a disability just as we would if Robbie had been born to us. We had our period of denial and hope that he would 'catch up' after adoption, went through a period of sadness and loss, and emerged with a characteristic determination to help him do the best he possibly can.

We were fortunate in having a determinedly inclusive primary school at the top of our road. Robbie joined his new sister at her school, welcomed and supported by the community. The children shared experiences as other siblings do and enjoyed a deep sense of security. Families who knew Robbie then still look out for him in the neighbourhood and have come to his rescue several times. The police once questioned Robbie while he was waiting outside a house for a friend. Not just one but two parents who knew him from school rang us to say they had seen what was going on, challenged the police, explained that Robbie should not be questioned without an adult and reassured him he was not about to be sent to jail.

'Differences' became more problematic at secondary school. For Robbie, the daily challenges of coping at our local comprehensive became daily traumas. 'Cussing' mothers was a source of constant friction and Robbie had his birth mother, foster mother and me to defend. Eleven-year-olds in inner London move to many different schools and Robbie lost the protection of boys who knew him and his family. Seeking friendship but lacking skills, he became isolated with one or two boys who themselves had marked emotional and behavioural needs. Girls from his primary schools befriended him but this became difficult as the gender divide began. Perhaps in desperation, Robbie began to draw on his sense of being 'different' as a way of seeking much needed care. At one point he told his year head that he was particularly upset because he had 'just' found out he was adopted. A few weeks later we were offered commiseration about the cancer Robbie had convinced the staff he had just been diagnosed as having.

We moved Robbie to a special school which Mark knew well as a psychologist. It happens to be near the school he attended briefly before coming to live with us. Robbie has made friends, been much happier, experienced greater success, gained in independence and managed public transport. But returning to the place where he and his siblings once lived together, every day, has raised painful questions for him.

Our daughter found secondary school difficult too. Julia found pupils increasingly dividing into social subgroups by class or ethnic minority heritage, and expressed her need for parents of the same ethnic background as herself to help her deal with racism at school and on the streets. She felt everyone expected her to be 'just' a white middle-class girl following predetermined pathways. She was intensely aware of inequalities, typified by Robbie's and her own birth families, and at the same time was surrounded by messages emphasising competition, materialism and elitism. Not being sure about who she was made it especially difficult to decide what she might want to be. Such concerns are not, of course, the sole province of adopted children and their parents, as friends and family constantly remind us when we turn to them for advice and support.

Nineteen years later we feel as we did at the outset, that a positive stance towards adoption is preferable for children and parents to a grudging, fundamentally negative one. Of course, it would be better if all families could care for their children and if in-country adoption was available for every child who required adoption. Of course, potential adopters should be carefully vetted and children matched to families as closely as possible. Of course, legal proceedings should protect the rights of children and parents. But for our two children at least, adoption secured them basic rights of health, education and family support, which it is not at all clear any available alternatives would have been able to provide.

Our children however still encounter a 'poor you' response when they explain they are adopted, especially from young people. Perhaps such comments echo some of the official and unofficial views about adoption held in recent years. The notion that best policy, even with severely dysfunctional families, is to leave children with birth parents as long as possible implies that if you end up being adopted, things in your family must have been really bad. Added to this may be unspoken prejudices, which my parents' generation felt more able to express, about the possible effects of 'bad blood' or 'poor stock' on a child. It does not seem helpful for children such as ours to be considered 'unlucky' to be adopted, even though we may wish to acknowledge the sadness and loss involved.

Similarly, we welcome moves to reduce the time children wait before being adopted. For a child like Robbie, optimum nutrition and health care, emotional security and appropriate stimulation during his first six years would have made a significant difference to his intellectual and emotional development. Certainly for his two younger siblings, removal from their birth family and placement with their permanent family more quickly, seems to have been for the good.

Families adopting across cultures need positive support not reluctant compliance with the legal processes. In the overwhelming majority of cases, once children are in the UK, they will stay. In partnership with the voluntary sector, parents could be helped to meet others who have adopted from overseas, establishing links to help them through the difficulties they will face at a later stage.

We also support moves to improve adoption leave and provide adoption allowances for families taking on children like Robbie. It is important that paid adoption leave applies not just to children under school age. Robbie was six when he came to us and had a term at home before beginning school, but we needed time and emotional energy to adjust as a family, not simply to take care of Robbie during the school day.

Being paid a generous adoption allowance for Robbie has been tremendously helpful. We decided early on that one of us would always work part time so as to be available at the end of the school day, to deal with visits to school, and sort out special medical and educational needs as they arose. We have been able to meet Robbie's needs and afford holidays and activities to keep us all sane, especially at difficult times.

The welcome drive to promote inclusion in schools makes it more likely that adopted older children will be supported to join siblings and neighbours in their local school. On the other hand, plans for more specialist, and by implication, more selective, secondary schools will not help families adopting older children or those with special needs. Local authorities may need to help meet costs of extra tuition or alternative schooling if local schools prove unable to meet a child's needs.

Adoption has been a positive experience for our children and for us, though it has never been without its difficulties and challenges. Our children are different, racially and culturally, from each other, and different again, in those respects, from us. Each of us is an individual. There is much that can be done, as I have stated, to make the adoption process positive and its outcomes beneficial. But at the end of the day, children and parents are individuals and services need to be planned around that inescapable fact.

22

BEING TRANSRACIALLY ADOPTED: WHAT IT'S REALLY LIKE IN THE UK

Julia Austin

People find out quickly that I'm adopted. This is either because I am very open with the fact – adopt pride? – or they look at my parents – I am from the island of Java whilst my parents are white and hail from Birmingham. What follows is always the same: 'Does that make you sad?' I continue with my much-repeated pro-adoption speech: 'Adoption means that the new parents will really want the child whereas in lots of natural families this is not necessarily the case'. I also mention that my parents have always been open about my adoption, there were no secrets. I might also add that I was adopted at three days old – no painful years or even months in care or foster homes. They ask if I will try to find my first family. They ask if I miss my 'mum'. It seems that I am put on trial, forced to argue my case. It is crucially important that I win because otherwise I will be an object of pity. Yet other such objects of pity, like blind or disabled people, are not usually exposed to similar questioning. Sometimes people even feel able to confide in me that they'd feel horrible if they were adopted. You begin to suspect you're a bit like the Elephant Man after that. What can you say? After all, any positive point about adoption simply translates as denial. My therapist seemed to believe that the root of my problems lay in the fact that I refused to stay with the pain of rejection by my first mother. Don't get your hopes up – there's no light at the end of the tunnel, there's nothing you can do other than accept that you're a reject. (It's no wonder The Raggy Dolls theme tune – 'Look who's in the reject bin' – was my favourite children's programme.) I had several therapists, during a stormy adolescence, two secondary schools which didn't work out, and finally a boarding school in Bath which helped me to turn my life around. I ran away from school, got depressed, and couldn't get on with my peers, especially girls. I also modelled professionally for a time when I was sixteen, and had some wild times. I still don't know what it was all about. Perhaps it was just a heightened form of teenage angst. I strongly believe my grim period was unrelated to being adopted. I'm glad it's over now.

Despite everyone asking as many questions as possible, they never ask what it feels like to be a different colour from my parents. Ironically, the area which has caused me considerable grief is quickly interpreted as a modern fairytale. Don't get me wrong, I would be stupid not to realise that I am very lucky to have been brought to England from the slums of Jakarta, it's just that the consequences of this process seem to have been wrapped in a chocolate-box veneer. I think this is mainly because it's my mother who relates the tale of 'how I came to be an Austin' and she has not been on the receiving end of racial identity issues. My parents have never had to experience the feelings I get when we have a pub lunch in the countryside. They simply don't have to deal with the stares that have sometimes meant I cannot enjoy the meal. When I tell them, they say that this is paranoia, that the stares are not hostile but simply due to my stunning exotic beauty (mother's at the wishful thinking game again). It's as though for everybody else, the story ends 'happily ever after' at the point of English arrival. I am not trying to suggest that I have had to endure a lot of racial abuse but I do have to contend with a lot of narrow-minded thinking and racial stereotyping. And unlike ethnic minority families, I do not have a mother, father or sibling with whom I can share similar experiences. Nor do I have family that gives me a strong sense of my own ethnic culture. And herein lies the confusion because essentially, you see, I am a white middle class English girl and not an Indonesian. Yet to just look at me, you'd have one bona fide ethnic minority (ethnic monitoring group: South East Asian Other).

The real trial for me of transracial adoption therefore has been a problem of physical appearance. I grew up with Barbie and the twins from Sweet Valley High as the ultimate role models of physical desirability. The images retain their hold over me to this day. Deeply ingrained in my psyche is the 'ideal woman', in other words cascading blonde locks, sparkling sea-blue eyes and mountainous breasts. My role models were whacky white actresses like Juliette Lewis and Heather Graham, not glamorous South East Asian superstars like Vanessa Mae or Lucy Liu. Equally ingrained is the knowledge that I fail miserably on all three counts. And equally imprinted is the notion that looks are everything. Now my parents will interject at this point, reminding me that they inundated my childhood with alternative views and that I have chosen to accept Plastic America. But the truth of the matter is that they simply cannot relate, not having grown up with the same pressures and the same level of non-conformity. Though they may have tried, *Clever Gretchen and other forgotten tales* just didn't have the same impact as Disney's *Cinderella* or *Sleeping beauty*. All I ever wanted was Barbie and to have a Kid's Meal at McDonald's. But can this be considered even remotely surprising in the face of such marketing giants? These very companies were, after all, paramount, if not in total control of my developing self-image.

So, in response to my parents intervention concerning 'choice', I would say that they chose to flout convention, which resulted in them heading off to Java and returning with somebody who would – without any choice in the matter whatsoever – be forced to tackle all these issues head on.

Aside from the issue of how I see myself, I also have to contend with other people's perceptions of me based on my ethnic appearance. At school I was painfully aware of how my white middle-class contemporaries judged and viewed ethnic minorities. Hierarchies were formed according to race and I found that different socio-economic situations had different pecking orders. At my North London private school, because there was a high percentage of rich Indians, being Indian was considered 'acceptable', whereas at my North London state school they were at the bottom of the heap. Interestingly, being 'black' was considered as acceptable as white in terms of street credibility. (In terms of actual acceptance – as intellectual and social equals – I sadly do not think the same can be said.) Attending boarding school in Bath was by far the most disturbing of all my experiences. All the white kids stayed in one group, all the black kids played basketball and all the Cantonese kids sat and ate noodles together. Nobody mixed. Nobody made the time to break the stereotypes. Within the teaching staff and the institution itself I felt a strong sense that the ethnic minority groups were viewed as second-class citizens. My friends were from the white middle class but as an additional plus, the Cantonese kids were also interested in befriending me. On the other hand, there were many painful times for me when my white contemporaries made racist jokes and remarks. I couldn't laugh because they were referring to people like me, weren't they? But then, if I really wasn't 'white middle class', surely I wouldn't be privy to such insider 'jokes'?

Stereotyping people according to skin colour is evident when people look at the Austin family. When we went to Egypt on holiday, the Egyptians assumed I must be the family servant. When a white friend accompanied us on a family outing, she was let in on the family ticket while I got given the 'friend' pass. My brother is also adopted but actually looks as if he could be the child of mum and dad. I do not tend to feel antagonism towards my brother for not understanding my 'otherness' because he has to cope with his own distinctness – marked learning difficulties. He is going his own way like me, but not in the same direction. Perhaps this fact has in a sense saved me from feeling excluded from the wider family, since the more conservative relatives have found it harder to accept him. I often feel like the black sheep of the family but this has more to do with what I choose to do rather than what I look like or where I come from.

In terms of my relationship with my parents, coming from Indonesia is for them I think a very positive thing. My parents lived in Indonesia for three years and I know that the memories from that time are some of the best of their lives. I am, in a way, a living souvenir of this great period. From the age of five to when I was fifteen, I was a member of the South Bank Youth

Gamelan group. This was beneficial to everyone as it kept alive a love for my country and its culture. The fact of being adopted, as I have mentioned, does not seem to have been especially hard for me. My parents had tried for a decade to have a child of their own and when they got me it was as though I was the long awaited special one. Rather, difficulties arose from being brought up as 'the special one' rather than feeling the unloved and unwanted one. The resulting bond between my parents and myself is very strong and I know that we are closer than many families. This has obviously been of tremendous value to me and all three of us know that I would be lost without them. They are my family, and I hardly ever think about being adopted.

The combination of closeness and security alongside a sense of being 'special' in some ways has enabled me to take daring decisions about the way I want to lead my life. I am strong-willed, I admit, and hard to handle at times, but I am intensely ambitious and have a great desire to succeed in what ever I end up doing. At the moment I have decided to turn down my place at university to see if I can become an actress. I like to think of myself as a Renaissance woman, able in the future to act, write and be really creative. One of the positive aspects for me of transracial adoption is that it has allowed me to have more freedom and choice and that people do not expect me to conform. I do not have a clue what the future holds and that is the beauty of it – what lies ahead is my blank page and I'm going to fill it exactly how I want.

23

FROM CHINA WITH LOVE

Angela Knight

When John and I moved from London to the Berkshire countryside with our newborn daughter, Sasha, twelve years ago, we never thought that one day our efforts to have another child would take us on an emotional roller coaster through the despair of IVF and a two-and-a-half-year journey meandering through the protracted bureaucracy of the adoption system. Or that the red tape would open doors to a fascinating, new culture, new friends and eventually lead us to the other side of the world.

Sasha's first summer was idyllic, we had a small cottage with a large, rambling English country garden, croquet lawn and beautiful views of the Downs beyond. I remember Sasha lying in her pram under ancient apple trees swathed in clematis or us sitting on an old swing breathing in the scent of azaleas.

We were in our late thirties and in a hurry to have another child. As Sasha grew older she would cry every time one of her friends had a new sister. But after three IVF attempts and a major operation I told her she wasn't likely to have a sister. Adoption had crossed our minds, but I was told there were no babies available and we were too old to adopt in this country as we were over 35. It was at the time of the war in Bosnia, and I rang a charity helping babies orphaned by the war but was told that adoption would definitely not be an option because the orphans needed to stay in their own culture. I rang British Agencies for Adoption and Fostering several times and left messages on an answerphone. Some time later I was advised to contact my local authority. As I lived on the border of three counties it was difficult to know which one to contact and when I did track down someone, I didn't make any headway. I heard about OASIS (Overseas Adoption Services Information and Support), a voluntary adoption organisation which sent me information about the different adoption regulations around the world. I pored over them and filed them away.

By this time we had moved to a larger house complete with paddocks and chickens. We couldn't have been happier as a family of three and we relished Sasha's progress every day. Having been a teacher in the East End of London and seen deprivation and poverty, I felt we should share what we had with children who weren't so fortunate. And so, along the twisty, windy route of adoption we enquired about fostering or offering a deprived child a holiday in our home. John, understandably had reservations about what effect this might have on Sasha so, in the end, despite attending a presentation on fostering and being interviewed to take a child during the holidays, we didn't go ahead with either possibility.

Then I happened to read in the paper about a Channel 4 documentary called *The dying rooms*. It took a harrowing look at China's orphanages, packed with abandoned baby girls because of that country's one child per family policy. It struck a chord and seemed to be the answer to our prayers, on top of which we would be saving a life. This made me all the more determined.

With the help of OASIS I got in touch with others who had adopted from China and tracked down the Brooke family, who were one of the first to do this. They came all the way from Bristol with their daughters Georgina, aged five, and three-year-old Victoria, who both came from China, and talked us through the process. The system hinged on a home study report, compiled by a social worker. The report would be put before a panel of experts to decide whether or not we were suitable parents to adopt. It cost from £1,100–£6,000 as there was no limit to what an authority could charge.

Our local social services director was very helpful and recommended we contact the Oxford Diocesan Council for Social Work in Reading (now called PACT), one of two independent organisations in the country (the other is Childlink), whose home studies are recognised by the Department of Health. I was worried about how long it would take because by now we were forty somethings. The cost was another concern so we opened a China Fund savings account.

After an interview in November 1995 with the director of the ODCSW I felt elated, we were on our way to passing GO – as long as we paid £2,200 and filled in the first of what were to seem hundreds of forms. Patience is an asset but perseverance a necessity as there were countless occasions when we waited for replies or documents.

We all had to have thorough medicals. I couldn't help thinking that ordinary parents didn't have to do this or the home study, they just went ahead and produced babies. Among other things my doctor had to check for were varicose veins. Anyone would have thought I was going to give birth to the baby myself.

In the New Year of 1996 Hilary, our social worker, arrived to meet us. I had been frantically tidying the house when a friend who had an adopted daughter from Brazil advised me not to make the place too tidy and to scatter toys around. Her seven visits would last three hours each among a debris of toys. We found her down to earth and professional and felt she was sympathetic, although she hadn't been involved with an adoption from China before. She would leave us with written questions about our own upbringing, education, employment, religious beliefs, ideas on marriage and parenting and was quite intense. On one visit she had to interview Sasha, who was six at the time and we held our breaths when she was asked what her Mummy and Daddy were like. To get to know her, Hilary asked Sasha to take her on a guided tour of our house. From our answers Hilary compiled a comprehensive report (Form F) on us.

On our wedding anniversary in the Spring our spirits plummeted. We learnt that the Chinese authorities now required parents who already had children to adopt a child with special needs like a cleft palate, hare-lip, hole in the heart, club foot or birth mark.

In the meantime, we had to attend workshops dealing with adopting a child from another race and were able to meet others in the same boat; it was thought provoking and there was a good feeling of camaraderie within the group. However, one of the talks was given by a woman who had worked in a Chinese orphanage. She told us that if we didn't accept a child offered to us, it would certainly die.

By April, the processing of applications to adopt slowed down in China and Hilary still had to interview two of our referees before our report went to the adoption panel. In May though, there were lovely baby clothes in the sales, but I was unable to buy anything because I didn't know what age our child would be. To cheer myself up I bought a pink piglet for her. But making the slightest preparation for her arrival made me superstitious as we found we slid down more snakes than climbed ladders in this waiting game.

There were moments of intense frustration when, for example, I was checking our home study report and noticed it stated that we were prepared to accept a child over 18 months and one which had been sexually and physically abused or disabled. I suggested this should be changed because translated into Chinese, it could be misinterpreted as a request. Hilary said as we were likely to get an older child the panel would not pass us unless we put this in. It seemed like a Catch 22 situation but we compromised and changed it, adding a paragraph which stated that obviously we would not know our child's background, she may have been abused and we were prepared to take that risk and although we may be offered a child with a minor disability, we would prefer a healthy infant.

In the summer we heard that we had passed the home study. It was a huge relief. Even though we were parents already, an anonymous group of people could have stopped us giving a child a home and a future. It was a hot, sunny afternoon, Sasha and I were playing in the garden. I decided not to tell her because I thought we probably wouldn't be going to China until Christmas which was a long way off. Later that evening, John and I watched the mayflies on the pond and wondered whether the baby we would be offered had been born.

Our progress took a nose dive sometime later. We had been watching a moving programme about a couple whose baby had died. They had wanted to adopt but had failed their home study. At that moment Hilary rang to say that the Department of Health had deferred our application and wanted two further references.

As the days passed, it was a case of one step forward, two steps back. In China, the Ministry of Justice had combined with the Civil Affairs Department and there was said to be a backlog of 600 adoption applications. We were told to get documents such as passports, birth certificates, marriage certificates, financial statements, and Sasha's Medical notarised. Our file was forwarded by the Department of Health and sent to Beijing in August 1996.

In November we heard that our file had joined the backlog with the others and we would not hear anything before March 1997. I was worried that as time went on we would drop out mainly because we weren't getting any younger. The waiting was proving too much for Sasha; she told me that she would prefer us to adopt a caravan rather than a baby.

Three things kept us going: the quarterly newsletter from OASIS, hearing that others had been matched with their babies, and asking a sympathetic Chinese man, Yao Hu, to ring Beijing and find out at what stage our file was. Christmas came and went with no news from China and in the New Year we sent £800 to the Chinese authorities for translation costs. I visited the January Sales and saw all the toys and baby clothes and felt gloomy. But punctuating these low points there was usually news of others who had heard. Some friends locally had been matched, they had no children and heard the news on a flight to New York. They had waited 18 months and said it was like waking up again after being drugged for ages. The waiting and not knowing was excruciatingly numbing for us but it must have been worse for those without children.

To keep our spirits up a group of us met at a Chinese restaurant, the Chef Imperial in Woodstock, for the Chinese New Year. We were all excited about the prospect of hearing. We talked about being in China – perhaps in May? But in the spring we heard that special needs cases were taking longer. I was still concerned about what we would be offered in the way of a minor handicap and couldn't bear to think of rejecting a baby after all this. In June, the first of our group to hear went out to China to collect their 17-month-old daughter, Grace. Then in August, another friend was matched with 14-month-old, Isabel Fu Ming. It was getting exciting knowing the wheels were grinding, albeit at a snail's pace.

In the autumn, the experience of being in suspended animation, not being able to plan ahead, weighed heavily on me and I thought that maybe we would give up. On the spur of the moment I invited a friend over with her new Chinese baby, Amy. She was simply gorgeous and charmed us both; we were on track again.

Despite the agony of waiting for a letter to arrive from the Department of Health, I refrained from badgering the department by phone to check our progress but, on the advice of a friend, on 1 October 1997 I rang. To my surprise, I was told that a list of 13 names had been received and it was now being translated. On further checking I was told that we had been matched with a baby called Wang Ze Rong, who had been born in February. Hot tears streamed down my face in relief that we had at last heard, but even more importantly we could focus our thoughts on a child who was waiting for us to come to her thousands of miles away.

A week later we received a medical report for a baby who was now called She Shajiang, born 28 March 1997. It was in Chinese and I had no idea what it said. My husband was playing badminton that evening and knowing I couldn't look at those indecipherable squiggles all night, I rushed down to a local Chinese restaurant. There I was offered jasmine tea and told that our baby was a girl and had an ulcer on her left cornea. I was euphoric.

The next day, I tracked down a Chinese doctor in this country who had worked in Chinese orphanages. He told me that he gave the medical two out of ten and that our daughter could go blind or be blind because of the conditions in the orphanage. Could I take on a child blind in one eye, I asked myself? I took a chance and rang the China Women's Travel Agency in Beijing to see if they could find out how She Shajiang was doing. They were very helpful. A day later I rang again and they told me that she was well and the eye had healed. The news was like a miracle and I was overcome with relief. I somehow knew everything would be alright. The next day we received a small colour photograph of her, she was beautiful and she was smiling. I bonded with her in seconds! As the news spread to friends I felt I was floating on a wave of euphoria. I kept telling She Shajiang to hold on, we would be coming to fetch her soon. There were visas to apply for and a nerve-wracking wait for an invitation from the Chinese authorities to travel to China. This could have taken up to six months but arrived only two weeks later.

In November I received a fax that She Shajiang weighed only 4.5kg (10lb), at least I now knew what size clothes to take – very small and a friend lent me a bag full of tiny babygros. As 19 November, our departure date, grew nearer I thought I would burst with happiness, Sasha was excited and John was busy sorting out our travel arrangements. The fact that we were going to China seemed so unreal after all the waiting. We couldn't wait to meet She Shajiang and bring her home.

In retrospect, the worst time for all of us, particularly Sasha, was when, two months later, we arrived in China. Sasha found the food strange and the imminent arrival of a stranger, whom we might love more than her, very distressing. Trying to give her the same amount of attention as she was used to and caring for a new baby was difficult for me practically and emotionally. John gave Sasha his undivided attention which made me feel as if we had divided into two as a family. It was upsetting but somehow we came through it with a lot of effort and adjustment on all sides. Tamzin, as we had now renamed She Shajiang, was unwell on the 14-hour flight back so that arriving home was a wonderful moment. The house was warm and welcoming. The girls' rooms had been decorated while we were away. Sasha was over the moon and I put Tamzin in her cot for the first time. She seemed to accept this as home and us as her family and we've never looked back. Having got over the jetlag and Christmas festivities, Tamzin settled in very quickly. She smiles endlessly at us and has learnt to wave. She adores Sasha and it is touching to see them play together. She is bright and alert and loves her food, usually holding it in both hands, then looking at her hands, then at us, then at her hands, then at us, before putting the food in her mouth. She is gaining over a pound a week and sleeping through the night. Tamzin is developing well and has now surprised us by walking. I am still euphoric, we could not have wished for a better baby and I am thankful that we were unsuccessful with IVF otherwise we would never have known her.

Our only concern has been to make sure Sasha receives as much love and attention so that she doesn't feel she has been displaced. She told us that it's different now Tamzin is here, but she's glad she's got a sister and she is very attentive to her. At Christmas, our relatives naturally focused on the new baby but we are fortunate that Sasha expresses herself and we can discuss her feelings. We feel lucky to have two wonderful daughters, one blonde the other dark. John is enchanted by Tamzin and will now admit that he had reservations about adopting because he thought we were happy as a threesome and did not want to spoil that. But he is now so pleased that we did. We feel it has worked out better than we ever dared hope.

Four years later we are very lucky – we have two wonderful daughters who love each other. Tamzin has just started school with Sasha and adores following in her footsteps. Sasha in turn is very loving and keeps an eye on her little sister. Tamzin is very demonstrative and radiates joy, she has a huge smile and is extremely affectionate. When I pick her up from school she runs towards me, arms outstretched, socks at half mast, paint smudging her cheeks calling: 'Mummy, mummy! I love you!' Over the years we have tried to give the girls the same amount of love and attention and both children, we think, feel very loved and secure. The only residue of Tamzin's previous life is night terrors, each one extremely distressing to witness. I know that she is back in the orphanage from the way that her legs are stretched out straight in front of her and her body is rigid, her eyes stare angrily into the dark and she beats her fist in desperation crying furiously. Fortunately, these are occurring less and less.

I was surprised to hear recently that PACT is no longer allowing couples with a birth child to adopt because 20 per cent of these adoptions are said to break down. We are so thankful that Tamzin is part of our family, it would not be the same without her and we have to admit that it is not she who is the lucky one, it is us.

This year was the seventh time we have celebrated the Chinese New Year with other families who have adopted children from China. We celebrate their birthdays and have reunions so that these Chinese children with dark hair and Chinese eyes will have friends who look like them and, in the future, can share any problems and worries they may have. Perhaps one day when Tamzin has grown up, she will return to China and trace her origins. But we hope that she will always know where her home is.

24

REJECTION AND
ACCEPTANCE

Sheena and Donald Macrae

In September 1996 we began our home study assessment to adopt a child from China. We had an immediate rapport with our caseworker, and were delighted to accept her challenge to provide written responses to some of the sections in her report. I took up a second challenge of working as an unpaid classroom assistant in a local school to show willing toward gaining hands-on experience with very young children.

Things proceeded quickly. The assessment was completed in November; the second opinion visit also approved us, and we went to our local adoption panel on 5 December with strong caseworker support.

It was a total shock, then, when our caseworker phoned late on the afternoon of the day that the panel met to say that it had rejected our application. We were devastated and also angry. Our caseworker and the team leader were also taken aback and very sympathetic to our grief and despair. They had been sure that we would have passed through with ease. They arranged to meet us within a few days to support and help with our feelings of anger and disbelief, to discuss the panel's reasoning, and to discuss the appeal that they strongly urged we make.

The panel had rejected us on four grounds. The first was that we had not shown evidence of enough cultural sensitivity to the needs of a child adopted from abroad. Second, the panel believed that my 'history of anxiety' could make me unable to cope with the adoption process and being an adoptive parent. Third, our expectations of children likely to be placed were said to be unrealistic, and we would be unable to balance this because we would invest too much in the child. Last, the panel believed that we had a number of unresolved issues in our own experiences of being parented; it felt that adoption could set off these unresolved problems.

It seemed that rather than having presented a good home study, we were being questioned to the very core of our own judgement about ourselves. The home study had been a very personal and deeply intensive period, and it felt very bad indeed to have these questions asked. It was all the worse because we had written some of the responses. We wished – in a sense – that our caseworker had not been so impressed with us that she had let us do this.

At the meeting with the caseworker, the team leader also attended. She was very careful to say that until she had met us in person to conduct the second opinion visit, she had had serious qualms about our being down-to-earth-enough people to make good parents. She explained that she felt that our contribution to the home study had not helped her come to see us as rounded people. More, she felt, our responses were a literary exercise designed to persuade by argument, rather than present people who could cope and care.

I was rocked to the core, but in one sense I could not take it personally. I found that I was seeking very hard to feel more than understand what the panel had said and what the team leader was now saying. I found it hard though. I felt very hurt that my health and personality were being questioned when my chronic illness had forced me in dealing openly with both.

My husband took it personally straightaway; he reckoned it was a personal and insulting attack. However, our common response was to deal with the questions, reassert ourselves and try to convince the panel we were people who could cope and could deal with children.

The team leader told us we should appeal, and an appeal was lodged and set for five weeks later. She also urged that we should attend personally. That way the panel would see us as she had found us. And she said she thought we were thoughtful rather than cerebral! She was sure that this personal appearance would be the key to the appeal's success. We agreed. Our defence would be that we were rounded and thoughtful people.

We decided that although writing parts of the home study had not helped us before, we would still present our case to the panel by letter. We wanted to do this because we were aware that our appearance at the appeal could not guarantee that we would be able to get our case across. The panel could take off in new directions. And they did.

Because the time between the panel decision and the appeal was over Christmas and New Year, we had to work hard to garner support. On the other hand, time dragged over the holiday period. We had hoped to spend this Christmas anticipating future Christmases with children. The future now looked very bleak.

Dealing with the medical issue of my 'history of anxiety' was relatively straightforward. I had a consultation with my GP; he had done the adoption medical which the panel had taken issue with. He was astounded; he had made a very firm recommendation that I would make a good adoptive parent. He readily agreed to write a letter to the adoption team's medical adviser detailing how in fact I had dealt with and deal with my chronic illness, and how I had dealt with the anxiety that arose round it when I had a very serious operation in 1983. He and I agree that when one has a chronic illness it is very important to have a good and close relationship with the medical services (I do) and to be proactive when trouble arises (I am). That done, we felt there was no more we could do to clarify this issue.

Dealing with the problems of being insensitive to cultural needs made us cross. We had presented a good deal in the home study to show how we would ensure the child grew up at ease with her ethnic origins. We asserted we had stated this, and went on to present a little more. We have always felt that being Scots living in England gives a tiny taste of being 'different'. We said that we would always be sensitive to any feelings that the child had of difference, would ensure she had access to what of her own culture is available here, and, more importantly, would return on regular trips to her country of birth.

We took more time to think very carefully about our so-called 'unreasonable expectations of the children likely to be placed' and of unresolved issues of our own childhoods being retriggered by the adoption and by becoming parents.

Regarding those 'unreasonable expectations', it seemed to us that the panel probably had seen us as narrowly academic in outlook or at least high-flying in jobs and with a more 'intellectual' perspective on life than many. And with this they probably felt we might be insensitive even to the needs of an average child. Thus, they probably considered we could not remotely cope with a child with post-institutional emotional and possibly cognitive loss. Having seen that this might have concerned the panel, there was little else we could do than to say we understood their concerns. However, we feel (and felt) that we do understand these needs – we read, attended seminars and talked with other parents who experience these problems. We could do little more than say we intended being proactive to the needs of a child who would arrive with loss. Understanding a personal loss makes for the understanding of it in others. We hoped to convince the panel we could handle our losses, and turn the understanding into a gain for the child.

The panel had said that it would be hard for us to achieve a balance in suiting the child and hoping she would in some way meet our aspirations. I personally found this a damning comment on my capacity to empathise with the needs of my child. However, I reminded myself that the panel's major considerations are with the needs of the child and, therefore, they were quite justified in having this concern.

Our answer was that expectations exist in every family, and children do not always arrive in the way birth parents hope. However, we were prepared to parent and learn for the child whatever the needs, and, again, being thinking and proactive would be more of a help than a hindrance. If help for post-institutional problems arose, we would search till the child received the help needed.

The question of unresolved issues about our own parenting being re-opened by adopting was challenging. However, it seemed to us that the panel were being too harsh on us for dealing with the losses we felt we had experienced in our own childhoods (workaholic fathers (both of us), weak and doting mother (me)).

Again we understood that since the panel must be primarily concerned with the care of the child to be adopted, this concern was appropriate. Unfortunately, there are many people who become adoptive parents and have unresolved personal issues. This is unacceptable if they use their child to rework these issues. I know of parents who require behaviours of their children because they want a reward from the children for being 'saved' by them having adopted them.

This was not the case for us. We had hoped to show the panel that we understood problems of parenting through parenting which had not been perfect in our own cases. We felt and feel that this is actually a bonus. Understanding loss and mismanaged childhood situations and problems can help avoid a pattern developing from one generation to the next.

This was our case to the panel. We accepted that they were right in some way. When there is a crisis in family relations and the adult is thrown off balance, it takes control and hard work to avoid one's own mother's or father's reaction coming straight out. Such reactions are so deeply learned that they become almost instinct. In a crisis I can feel my mother's response coming back; it's hard to go a different way. And it's fair also to say that in reacting in this way, I now am very able to see with unblinkered eyes (that is, as a parent myself) where she was coming from when she dealt with me.

The day before the panel meeting on 16 January 1997, we shook all day. We were the last item on the agenda. I was so nervous that I realised that I had left the fridge door open just as we walked into the meeting, and I managed to blurt this out almost immediately. I froze. 'What an anxious idiot they must think I am, I quite prove their case', I thought. But they laughed with me, a lovely genuine supportive laugh, acknowledging the burden on us that day. And for us, things proceeded with ease and grace from there.

They gave us a hard time. They accepted my GP's apology for having misrepresented the depth of the anxiety I had faced over the major operation to forestall my chronic and life-threatening illness. However, they did pursue with great concentration how I would deal with further flare-ups of the condition when a child's needs had to be paramount. I was honest: I would be proactive, seek help, and rely on networks of support in the community, as well as in the home to support me. They approved of this.

They accepted our assertions about being culturally sensitive. I think they had to – we had quoted from a social services circular issued by the Department of Health in February 1996 and asserted that we had met the criterion that we had 'made reasonable attempts to acquaint [ourselves] with the history and culture of the country of choice so that [we could] provide information to the child about . . . background and the traditions of his or her country'. We had plainly done this and more.

Last, the panel listened with great concern to our statements regarding 'our expectations of the child' and the 'unresolved issues' about our own parenting but they gave us no clue as to whether or not they accepted what we said.

We received a telephone call that evening to say the panel had approved our application. There are no words to describe how we felt. Personally vindicated, maybe, but joyous at knowing we were indeed approved to go on to be parents. It was inexpressible.

Our papers went to the Department of Health for perusal before the certificate of eligibility to make an intercountry adoption was attached. We then found that the DoH was challenging us on new grounds: my husband's prior ulcer and high-flying career. This time, the panel, its medical adviser and our caseworkers all swung into action on our behalf and we were finally approved in April 1997.

We received our first daughter on 13 April 1998 from Shenzhen, China, and our second from Dianbai, also in Guangdong Province, on 23 December 2001. We go to China each year, we have some really superb friends in Shenzhen, we've done newspaper journalism within Guangdong Province, and the Chinese have acknowledged how good this feels to them given that most want to challenge about the politics of birth control and the politics of children living in orphanages. I feel an honorary Chinese through my girls!

In parenting these children and in what we went through we learned much. The panel was right to make its challenge and we grew personally through that. Whether I would say so with such certainty if we did not have the children is another matter. Anyway, I am very blessed in the children, and taxed to death on the issues that inter-country adoption brings. I am not super-mum, but I hope thinking-mum!

A panel must give priority to the needs of children. It hurts, though, to be rejected as not good enough even if this is salvaged later. Those that fail to win an appeal will need very careful counselling for this new blow and new loss.

25

ADOPTION PANELS

A critique from within

Chris Hanvey

Why have the workings of adoption panels received so little attention? At a time when the long-term placement of children has been so much in the spotlight this omission is both curious and troubling. While the Draft National Adoption Standards for England, Scotland and Wales (Department of Health, 2001) commented both on the renewed requirement to permit potential adoptive parents to attend adoption panels and, in Section F, on the streamlining of administrative procedures, there is little about how they function. Similarly, the BAAF Adoption and Fostering was quick to point out that, in the much-heralded Prime Minister's Review on Adoption (BAAF Adoption and Fostering, 2001), factual information relating to panels is sometimes inaccurate. Not only is it untrue to call them 'committees' of the local authority, but also the minimum membership is seven not six and elected councillors are not independent members. While BAAF's response argues that panels are under-resourced, there is no consideration of how panels should function nor of their suitability to match parents and children.

We might, then, turn to some findings from research and expect to see guidance on how panels function and what can be learnt from their current organisation. And yet, while *Adoption now: messages from research* (Parker, 1999) deals with adoption outcomes, the preparation and selection processes, legal and court proceedings and issues of organisation, it pays scant attention to the very body that makes any kind of outcome possible. Even more surprising is the way in which panels are treated in the Social Services Inspectorate's report, *For the children's sake: an SSI inspection of local authority adoption services* (Social Services Inspectorate, 1996).

This report deserves consideration, as it provides a pointer to the way central government regards the function of panels. Again, there is some consideration of the procedural issues, although, fortunately, the report does not make some of the factual mistakes of the Prime Minister's Review. Panels are non-executive bodies, accountable to social services committees, but not sub-committees of them. The report found that the training and induction of panel members was, euphemistically, 'generally modest' and that, in some localities, their understanding of the role and function of panels, themselves, was imperfect (9.9).

Nonetheless, most observed panels adopted a 'businesslike approach' (9.13), whatever this might mean, and panel members took their responsibilities seriously. More critically, 'some panels did not act as the shapers and arbiters of good practice their legislative role invites them to be' (9.35) and urged authorities to provide the necessary support to panel members. The report also recommended a 'wider understanding among staff and service users of panel roles and proceedings' (9.38), without struggling, itself, to define what these 'roles and proceedings' really are.

Interestingly, what has been written about panels tends to fall into one of two categories. Either it is highly critical of the workings of panels or it makes proposals for change at what can only be regarded as the edges. One example of the latter is the report *Action plan to improve adoption services* (British Agencies for Adoption and Fostering, 2000). This found that only about a half of adoption panels routinely reviewed children waiting for adoption and proposed that, as a matter of good practice, all panels should review children awaiting adoption, every six months.

As an example of the critical, Pennie (1993) described the 'spoken or unspoken reputations of panels' and of the necessity 'to undertake a child centred appraisal and evaluation of the information presented on each case and then use that as the basis of decisions'. Instead of this happening 'what you are likely to get is a panel member who won't approve an application because they [*sic*] don't think very rich/unemployed/income-supported families are suitable because of what they have/have not got'. This goes to the heart of this chapter, as does Pennie's assertion of 'opposing councillors playing out party political difficulties which have remote, if any connections with child care planning'. These are serious accusations and one might have expected to find them at the heart of either research into adoption or government recommendations on the way adoption services should operate. The exclusion of either personal or political agendas to the range of complex issues faced by panels is essential to their credibility and effectiveness.

What the research and literature on panels does show, in the last twenty years, is what might be regarded as tinkering with procedures. As one example of the way progress has, in some ways, been made, we find that less than twenty years ago the current debate was very much about whether adoptive parents saw reports submitted to panels! With admirable enlightenment, Smith acknowledged that 'some social workers felt that it was too difficult for them to share their interpretations and comments with the people about whom they were writing' but commendably added that this practice should be encouraged (Smith, 1984). Ten years later, BAAF was, to some extent, arguing against the proposed increase in independent members to a third, feeling that by doing so the professional voice would be diluted in panel deliberations (British Agencies for Adoption and Fostering, 1994).

There is, however, one issue that has come to preoccupy panels in recent years and can be seen as much more than tinkering at the edges. It is that of the representation of parents at panel meetings and their right to be heard directly. *Adoption and Fostering*, BAAF Adoption and Fostering's professional journal, has looked at the issue on several occasions, both describing a pilot project in Hertfordshire (Hender, 1994) and also looking at how the introduction of parallel planning might add a new challenge to individual representation (Pepys and Dix, 2000). Results from these experiments are generally positive, stressing the need for careful panel training and emphasising the way in which meeting birth parents, for example, tended to balance the less positive comments in the Form E.[1] There would inevitably be an opportunity for deliberation without the parents being present, and specific issues of birth parents being invited to present their views on a plan for adoption before the courts have reached their decisions. However, this new spirit of openness which, in another context Smith (1994) was encouraging, has assisted in both the quality and transparency of panel proceedings.

It is hoped that the above demonstrates that the working of adoption panels has seldom been given the consideration that it deserves. Such an omission is like looking at the criminal justice system without examining the contribution made by magistrates' courts. Since, for example, approvals and matchings have to go through panels and given the increased scrutiny that adoption has received in recent years, one is driven to ask why they are not seen as part of the root and branch review that controversies surrounding the whole process of adoption have precipitated.

What we do have are effective notes of guidance on the regulations, processes and good practice in adoption and permanence. BAAF Adoption and Fostering's *Effective panels* (Lord *et al.*, 2000) is an invaluable guide to procedures. It not only reminds panels that they largely make recommendations, and not decisions, but also defines the role of the agency decision maker; outlines the legal functions of the panel; looks at agency policy and practice issues; and also deals with, for example, matching and inter-country adoption. It is a useful review of the Adoption Agencies Regulations, 1983 and the Adoption Agencies and Children (Arrangements for Placement and Reviews) (Miscellaneous Amendments) Regulations, 1997. What the publication does not do – and by now it should be clear that none of the literature or research does – is to pose the fundamental question as to whether panels are the best means to reach decisions affecting children. The rest of the chapter will try to raise issues that are crucial to this question.

To a large extent the evidence needed to examine the above question has to be qualitative. Few, if any areas in social welfare can equal the complexity of approving adoptive parents or of matching them with children in need. Medicine rightly gains kudos from the life and death decisions that its practitioners sometimes have to make. Why is the matching of young lives with families, with whom they will be inextricably linked, not seen in the same light? And why, to repeat the opening statement of the chapter, are we not critically examining whether we have got the formal mechanisms for this matching right?

Those well versed in *Effective panels*, will be aware that all panels are a mix of social workers, lay members, advisers and elected members. The ethos, although not spelt out and certainly not questioned, is that by bringing together the ingredients of social workers well versed in adoption, those who have, by dint of experience, in some way encountered adoption, medical and legal advisers, and councillors, the result will be an admirable recipe. Furthermore, that this is the best method available for making sound decisions about children.

This ethos is both untested and unsound. First, there are few precedents for this kind of shared decision making. Child protection procedures, for example, frequently involve interdisciplinary case conferences as a way of decision making, but their professional membership does not extend to elected members or lay representation. Second, where is the research that decisions made in this kind of collective forum are in the best interests of children?

This latter point touches upon the views of Pennie, from her panel experience (Pennie, 1993). Given the large amount of interest and contro-versy that follows adoption, it is only natural that debates surrounding it should be the work of panels. Councillors bring specific perspectives, based on the political context within which they operate. Lay members, who have had either successful or unsuccessful experiences of adoption processes, will bring another perspective. Social workers may well be influenced by specific 'fashions' within adoption practice. The response might then be: 'Well, what is wrong with this? Surely this makes for a good well-rounded debate, where a number of viewpoints can be expressed?' The argument against this is twofold. First, are the over-riding factors necessary to good decision making based on personal views or prejudices or on verifiable evidence? Second, this kind of decision making can lead to consensus by compromise, where compromise itself is an enemy of best practice.

But all of this may smack of another conspiracy against the laity: an exclu-sion of independent members in order to bolster the social work presence and to ensure that common sense views are replaced by professional fashion or prejudice. However, some of the most cogent arguments sometimes put forward in panel discussions are made by lay or elected members and some of the most unsound by social workers. The trouble is that panels often combine the worst elements of interviewing for professional jobs. Minds are quickly made up, evidence is replaced by prejudice and political agendas or turf wars, and personal scores get fought out in the context of seemingly rational debate.

Furthermore, with the changes that have taken place in social work education in recent years, it is doubtful if the training is equipped to furnish most panels with skilled professionals who possess both a good knowledge of child care and detailed acquaintance with the practice of adoption. It is unlikely that many of the social workers who present cases will have experienced many examples of adoption in their practice, nor have gained the wisdom that can only come by living through complex human problems in a sustained and directed way.

What then is the solution? If it is accepted that, at best, there is not firm evidence or research that panels do help to make the best decisions for children and, at worst, they prevent such good decisions, then a major review is necessary to look at the process. It is no longer good enough, despite publications such as *Effective panels*, to assume that better training or fine tuning of the regulations will put right the fundamental flaws of the present process. It is now necessary to look, in detail, at the nature of the decisions that panels make, the relationship between the agency decision maker and the panel itself, and whether panels impede or help good decision making. This, as a first step, is now absolutely essential.

The second action is both more fundamental and difficult to achieve. It is also easy to misinterpret. I argued earlier that I was not in favour of professionals making all of the decisions, given their current level of training and expertise. What I have been led to conclude is that unless we can produce highly skilled and valued practitioners with considerable child care experience, then the present situation will never improve for children. Although research into adoption panels has been woefully inadequate, we are gathering an increasingly large volume of literature on what works in adoption practice. It is this that should be at the heart of adoption decisions and not well meaning views or personal prejudice, however genuinely or forcefully felt. This would lead, eventually, to panels comprising skilled practitioners in law, medicine and child care, who come together to consider the best interests of children. It means an emphasis on evidence and on reaching 'good enough' decisions amidst the welter of evidence that children's lives inevitably bring.

Adoption remains at the core of that 'gift relationship' which Titmuss (1970) defined in relation to blood donors. When adoptive parents and children come together, for that blend of selfish and unselfish motives that are probably at the heart of all gift relationships, the effect can literally be transforming. We owe it to children in the care system, now and in the future, that this process is as efficient as we can possibly make it.

Note

1   Form E gives details of a child needing a family placement.

Chris Hanvey is director of operations at Barnardo's. The views in this chapter are, however, his own.

References

British Agencies for Adoption and Fostering (1994), Adoption panels: serving whose interests? (editorial), *Adoption and Fostering*, vol. 18, no. 3.

BAAF Adoption and Fostering (2000), *Action plan to improve adoption services*, London, BAAF Adoption and Fostering.

BAAF Adoption and Fostering (2001), *Prime Minister's review on adoption: responses to the consultation report from The Performance and Innovation Unit*, London, BAAF Adoption and Fostering.

Department of Health (2001), *Draft national adoption standards for England, Scotland and Wales*, London, Department of Health.

Hender, P. (1994), Applicants attending local authority adoption panels, *Adoption and Fostering*, 18(1).

Lord, J., Barker, S. and Cullen, D. (2000), *Effective panels: guidance on regulations, process and good practice in adoption and permanence panels*, London, BAAF Adoption and Fostering.

Parker, R. (ed.) (1999), *Adoption now: messages from research*, Chichester, John Wiley & Sons.

Pennie, P. (1993), Adoption panels: room for improvement, *Adoption and Fostering*, 17(2).

Pepys, S. and Dix, J. (2000), Inviting applicants, birth parents and young people to attend adoption panels: how it works in practice, *Adoption and Fostering*, Winter, 24(4).

Smith, C.R. (1984), *Adoption and fostering*, Basingstoke, Macmillan.

Social Services Inspectorate (1996), *For the children's sake: an SSI inspection of local authority adoption services*, London, Department of Health.

Titmuss, R. (1970), *The gift relationship: from human blood to social policy*, London, Allen & Unwin.

26

ADOPTION, RACE AND
IDENTITY

Anna Gupta

Academic writing, professional practice, media interest in adoption and race
and identity are dominated by the arguments surrounding same race and
transracial placements. The issues raised are some of the most contested and
polarised in the whole adoption debate. This chapter explores the complexities of the debate, by discussing the historical context, examining the
research and drawing conclusions for future practice.

Since the 1960s the placement needs of black children have attracted
considerable attention. Before the mid-1960s it was commonly accepted that
black children were not 'suitable' for adoption (Thoburn *et al.*, 2000). During
the 1960s, as the numbers of white babies for adoption decreased, black
babies slowly became viewed as acceptable for white childless couples to
adopt, usually as a last resort (Gill and Jackson, 1983; Barn *et al.*, 1997).
The British Adoption Project was established in the mid-1960s and was the
first significant attempt to place black children for adoption. The vast majority
of the children were placed with white families. This was seen at the time as
progressive and innovative social work practice reflecting a philosophical
approach which argued that racial assimilation was best achieved by the
placement of black children with white families (Small, 1986; Barn, 1999).
Transracial adoption was also advocated as a way of reducing the disproportionately high number of black children in residential care (Small, 1986).

Gradually in the 1970s the critics of transracial adoption were beginning
to make their views heard. The Soul Kids campaign of 1975 was the first
dedicated attempt to recruit black families for black children. In 1980 the
success of the New Black Families Unit in Lambeth challenged the argument
for transracial placements on the grounds of a lack of black families (Small,
1986). In the mid-1980s, the Association of Black Social Workers and Allied
Professionals launched a campaign opposing transracial adoptions. In addition, increasing numbers of black young people brought up in transracial
placements were talking of their struggles with identity confusion and alien-
ation (Black and In Care, 1984).

A highly polarised and heated debate followed. Supporters of transracial placements argued that children were being denied loving, permanent homes for political and ideological reasons (Dale, 1987), while supporters of same race placements contended that psychological and political concerns could not be separated when considering children's development of positive black identities (Maximé, 1986).

Since the late 1980s, increasing numbers of black children have been placed with black families (Waterhouse, 1997). The Children Act, 1989 requires that due consideration be given to the racial, cultural, religious and linguistic needs of children when decisions are being made about placements. However, critics (including the right-wing press) have continued to brand social workers supporting same race placements as too 'politically correct' and some New Labour politicians, in particular the former junior health minister Paul Boateng, have reasserted the colour-blind approach by emphasising 'love not colour'. The White Paper on Adoption (Department of Health, 2000a) advocates the placement of children with families who reflect their birth heritage. However, it also states that 'no child should be denied loving adoptive parents solely on the grounds that the child and parents do not share the same racial or cultural background'.

The placement of white children has rarely figured in the debate. Cheetham (1982), Rhodes (1992) and Flynn (2000) are among the small number of researchers who explore the placement of white children with black carers. Rhodes (1992) noted that even when the participating borough faced an acute shortage of white carers, they did not at any point consider the placement of white children with black carers. Flynn (2000) argues that 'for white children who have readily available positive role models, and do not experience racism, black carers can open up options for white children and be an additional valuable resource'.

Children have a range of complex developmental needs which must be met during different stages in their childhood to promote their welfare and enable optimal outcomes to be achieved. The promotion of a positive identity forms a core component of Department of Health guidance on the assessment of children's needs (Department of Health, 1995; Department of Health, 2000a). *A framework for the assessment of children in need and their families* (Department of Health, 2000a) states that identity concerns 'the child's growing sense of self as a separate and valued person'.

Within the research literature there has been much debate on the links between self-esteem and racial identity and the complex methodological issues associated with the evaluation of outcomes. Gill and Jackson (1983) concluded that the majority of transracial placements studied could be deemed as 'successful', although 'there was little evidence of a positive sense of racial identity'. Similarly, Tizard and Pheonix (1989) asserted that their research demonstrated that children can develop positive self-concepts in transracial placements, although many had negative feelings about their racial identity. Many proponents of same-race placements have criticised the perception by these and other authors that racial identity and self-concept are two distinct variables (Banks, 1992; Barn, 1999).

Over the past 10 years child welfare professionals' knowledge of, and requirement to promote opportunities for the positive identity development of children in need have increased. The Utting report states:

> A positive sense of identity, of being somebody, of belonging to oneself, is an inner strength which provides the strongest personal defence against harm. Helping children achieve that identity . . . ought to be the explicit objective of any organisation entrusted with the care of children. This sense of identity is derived from membership of family and other groups with similar values with which early life experience is shared. Detachment from family and culture plainly impairs its development; membership of a distinctive or disadvantaged community may compound the difficulties; in the case of black children, their situation is further aggravated by the pervasive effects of racism.
>
> (Utting, 1999)

Dutt and Phillips (2000) propose a model of understanding identity which includes group and individual identity and the relationship between identity and other aspects of children's development. Identity is presented as incorporating many different aspects including race, culture, gender, class, disability and sexuality. Both black and white children have racial identities, however as white is perceived as the norm, being black becomes defined as different. In a society like Britain, where racism is endemic (MacPherson, 1999), a black child will receive negative messages about being black and needs a positive internal model of identity to counteract these negative messages. Factors promoting positive identity include secure attachment relationships, racially aware carers and positive black role models. Black children growing up with insecurity, rejection, hostility and racially unaware carers will find it much harder to develop both a positive group and individual identity (Dutt and Phillips, 2000).

Advocates of same race placements argue that black families are more equipped to be able to provide children with an awareness of racism, an ability to deal positively with experiences of racism and offer a wider range of positive black role models (Small, 1986; Barn, 1999; Prevatt Goldstein and Spencer, 2000). A Department of Health-funded study concluded that:

> The race of parents has an important bearing on how they fulfil the specific parenting tasks of helping children develop a positive racial and cultural identity, and confronting racism. . . . From the interview data we conclude that the requirement in the Children Act, 1989 to

seek to place children with parents who can meet their identified needs as individuals, and who are of a similar cultural and ethnic background, provides a sound basis for policy.

(Thoburn *et al.*, 2000)

As mentioned earlier, a person's identity incorporates many different aspects. Black people in Britain come from many different cultural, linguistic and religious traditions, which when different from the dominant tradition may also be subjected to stereotyping and negative valuation (Dominelli, 1992). The provision of cultural, religious and linguistic continuity for children in substitute care is crucial for the development of a positive identity. A government circular to Local Authorities states that:

> Maintaining continuity of the heritage of their birth family in their day-to-day life is important to most children; it is a means of retaining knowledge of their identity and feeling that although they have left their birth family they have not abandoned important cultural, religious or linguistic values

(Department of Health, 1998)

Same race placements may offer opportunities for some continuity of cultural, religious and linguistic traditions. However, attention must be paid to understanding the child's heritage, including ascertaining the wishes and feelings of children and families, and avoiding stereotypical and superficial assessments. Richards and Ince's (2000) study into local authority services for looked-after children found that only 29 per cent of local authorities had mechanisms for ensuring that a child's needs in terms of ethnicity, culture, religion and language were met on a daily basis, with religion being given a very low priority. Hussain Sumpton (1999) uses the case example of an Indian Muslim boy being placed with an Indian Sikh family to illustrate the complexities of placing Asian children. For example, Ali did not eat pork, while his Sikh foster family ate pork, but not beef. They spoke different Asian languages, so were only able to communicate in English, a language Ali's mother was not able to speak fluently. The local authority had not addressed these issues and were 'surprised that the placement was disrupting; after all, he had been placed in an "Asian" family' (Hussain Sumpton, 1999).

While all children have access to the dominant (white) culture, regional, class and religious differences are often under recognised (see Garrett, 2000 for an examination of the placement of Irish children). Prevatt Goldstein and Spencer (2000) argue that issues of identity and self-esteem are 'both significant for all children and require a different emphasis in placement depending on the degree of racism and marginalisation experienced by the child's ethnic group'.

The delay some black children experience by waiting to be placed with a racially and culturally matched family has long been cited as a criticism of same race placement policies. Delay in placing children in permanent placements can have a negative impact on their development and the older the child the greater the likelihood of placement breakdown (Sellick and Thoburn, 1996). However, while it is clearly in all children's interests that appropriate placements are made with minimum delay, there is a risk that children's long-term needs for a positive identity and self-esteem may be compromised by rushed and inappropriate placements (Prevatt Goldstein and Spencer, 2000). Instead efforts could be better focused on the recruitment and support of carers from a range of racial, cultural, linguistic and religious backgrounds. In light of the MacPherson report (1999) agencies need also to examine the impact of institutional racism. Richards and Ince (2000) found that only 38 per cent of local authorities had a specific recruitment policy for black and other minority ethnic carers.

A number of elements of the White Paper (Department of Health, 2000) can be seen as positive developments for black children. 'Special guardianship' may encourage some minority ethnic communities who have religious and cultural difficulties with adoption as it is set out in law. The Adoption Register should also enable the sharing of information on available adoptive families.

However, where it is not possible to place a child in a same race placement within a reasonable time or because of other factors such as the strength of the attachment relationship with its present carers, the placement of siblings together or an inter-country adoption, specific interventions need to be considered. These include recruiting and supporting families who are able to demonstrate an understanding of the developmental needs of black children and an active understanding of racism and commitment to challenging racism and discrimination; and promote the child's access to cultural, religious and linguistic frameworks which will provide continuity for the child, preferably in a multiracial setting (Prevatt Goldstein and Spencer, 2000; Thoburn *et al.*, 2000).

Adopted children are some of the most vulnerable in our society. Any adoptive family must seek to promote a child's positive identity and self-concept. Increasingly over the past decade theoretical knowledge, research and legislation have supported the views that black families from a similar religious, cultural and linguistic background, who are assessed as able to meet a child's developmental needs, offer children the best opportunities for optimal development. However, proactive responses need to be taken by local authorities and other adoption agencies to recruit and support suitable families from a range of racial, linguistic, cultural backgrounds; professionals need to undertake detailed and holistic assessments of children's needs; and where a placement is unable to meet these needs attempts must be made to facilitate the child's development of a positive identity. An understanding of the needs of black children can also facilitate the promotion of the needs of children from other minority groups experiencing discrimination.

References

Banks, N. (1992), Techniques for direct identity work with black children, *Adoption and Fostering*, 16(3), 19–25.

Barn, R. (1999), Racial and ethnic identity, in R. Barn (ed.) *Working with black children and adolescents in need*, London, British Agencies for Adoption and Fostering.

Barn, R., Sinclair, R. and Ferdinand, D. (1997), *Acting on principle: an examination of race and ethnicity in social services provision for children and families*, London, British Agencies for Adoption and Fostering.

Black and In Care (1982), *Black and in care*, conference report, London, Blackrose Press.

Cheetham, J. (ed.) (1982), *Social work and ethnicity*, London, George Allen & Unwin.

Dale, D. (1987), *Denying homes to black children: Britain's new race adoption policies*, London, Social Affairs Unit.

Department of Health (1995), *Looking after children (LAC) materials*, London, HMSO.

Department of Health (1998), *Adoption: achieving the right balance*, Local Authority Circular (98)20, London, The Stationery Office.

Department of Health (2000a), *Adoption: a new approach*, London, The Stationery Office.

Department of Health (2000b), A *framework for the assessment of children in need and their families*, London, The Stationery Office.

Dominelli, L. (1992), An uncaring profession? An examination of racism in social work, in P. Braham, A. Rattansi, and R. Skellington (eds) *Racism and Antiracism*, London, Open University and Sage.

Dutt, R. and Phillips, M. (2000), Assessing black children in need and their families, in Department of Health (eds) *Assessing children in need and their families*, London, The Stationery Office.

Flynn, R. (2000), Black carers for white children: shifting the 'same-race' placement debate, *Adoption and Fostering*, 24, 1, 47–52.

Garrett, P.M. (2000), Responding to Irish 'invisibility': anti-discriminatory social work practice and the placement of Irish children in Britain, *Adoption and Fostering*, 24, 1, 23–33.

Gill, O. and Jackson, B. (1983), *Adoption and race*, London, Batsford/British Agencies for Adoption and Fostering.

Husain Sumpton, A. (1999), Communicating with and assessing black children, in R. Barn (ed.) *Working with black children and adolescents in need*, London, British Agencies for Adoption and Fostering.

MacPherson, W. (1999), *The Stephen Lawrence inquiry*, *Report of an inquiry*, London, The Stationery Office.

Maximé, J. (1986), Some psychological models of black self-concept, in S. Ahmed, J. Cheetham and J. Small (eds) *Social work with black children and their families*, London, Batsford/British Agencies for Adoption and Fostering.

Prevatt Goldstein, B. and Spencer, M. (2000), *'Race' and ethnicity*, London, BAAF Adoption and Fostering.

Rhodes, P. (1992), Racial matching, in *Fostering*, Aldershot, Avebury.

Richards, A. and Ince, L. (2000), *Overcoming obstacles: looked after children: quality services for black and minority ethnic children and their families*, London, Family Rights Group.

Sellick, C. and Thoburn, J. (1996), *What works in family placement?* Barkingside, Barnados'.

Small, J. (1986), Transracial placements: Conflicts and contradictions, in S. Ahmed, J. Cheetham and J. Small (eds) *Social work with black children and their families*, London, Batsford/British Agencies for Adoption and Fostering.

Thoburn, J., Norford, L. and Rashid, S. (2000), *Permanent family placement for children of minority ethnic origin*, London, Jessica Kingsley Publishers.

Tizard, B. and Phoenix, A. (1989), Black identity and transracial adoption, in *New Community*, 15(3), 427–37.

Utting, W. (1997), *People like us: the report of the review of safeguards for children living away from home*, London, The Stationery Office.

Waterhouse, S. (1997), *The organisation of fostering services: a study of arrangements for the delivery of fostering services in England*, London, National Foster Care Association.

Part V

THE FUTURE OF ADOPTION

INTRODUCTION

As the gap between rich and poor widened in the nineteenth century and a new middle class started to appear, children in the workhouses (whose numbers intriguingly equalled the number of children in care today at around 58,000) became more sought after. Various pressure groups like the National Committee for Promoting the Boarding-Out of Pauper Children, wanted to take girls out of the workhouses to train them as domestic servants. Following the loss of over 1,000,000 men in World War I, a generation of bereaved, childless women, for whom marrying again was often not an option, were keen to see an adoption law enacted, to satisfy their desire to bring up a child. While charity and compassion motivated some rescuers of poor children, children were mostly there to meet the needs of adults in one way or another. The economic worth of children had receded with rising incomes and standards of living and the coming of universal education. Children began to be seen more as individuals with their own needs and rights. A few generations later, towards the end of the twentieth century, the welfare of the child principle became the cornerstone of legislation concerning children and was famously enshrined in the Children Act, 1989. This effectively redefined adoption as no more and no less than the right of a child without a family to a safe and caring one.

Adoption continues to affect many thousands of people in the UK today. Most adoptions are happy and straightforward, founded on the ability of adopters to give the child a sense of identity and self-worth. But in other cases key human rights are being violated. A young woman known to one of the editors remains angry that her adoption by her aunt was kept a secret from her until she found out by chance when she was 26 years old. She felt her personal world was destroyed in a split-second. How will the breach of trust she experienced be resolved? Will she accept that the adults in her life did their best? She has a daughter. Will her sudden discovery affect how she parents her? Such potentially debilitating secrecy is much rarer than it was. However, even in today's spirit of greater openness which pervades adoption – often from the time of the adoption taking place through to the right by adopted adults to find their birth parents – these are private questions kept from public view, in households up and down the land. Pressure for less secrecy in adoptions remains important, as suppression of information can be damaging, the more so when family members collude in the denial. The American singer and songwriter, Suzanne Vega, a white American brought up to think of herself as Puerto Rican, described it as an 'otherness within the family' (*Guardian Weekend*, 6 October 2001). Others, like the comedian Jim Davidson, have expressed the same lifelong confusion about being brought up or adopted by close relatives without ever being properly told who your real mother and father are within an extended family. Jimmy Thomas, minister in the first Labour government, grew up believing that his mother was his sister, a by no means uncommon way in which, at one time – and may be even sometimes now – a child born to an unmarried daughter was absorbed into the family.

Adoptions within the family, though sometimes fraught, are easier compared with adoptions from care, where both the children and the adoption process are more tangled. Indeed, many children with more complex needs now available for adoption in the UK would have been placed in residential homes for their entire childhood as recently as 30 years ago, and would be deemed unadoptable in many parts of the world today. It is far from clear that enough skilled adopters, or indeed foster carers, can be found for British children in need over the next century. Despite the fact that 94 per cent of prospective adopters who go through the assessment process end up being approved, the drop out rate before then is enormous. It may well be that new residential care homes will need to be developed to look after the growing number of adolescents with persistent emotional and behavioural problems. This would require considerable capital and revenue investment, as well as going against the direction of contemporary child care policy, principles and research.

Despite its politicisation, a consensus about the way forward for adoption unites supporters and critics. For instance, following a harrowing series of films about children who wait far too long to be adopted, Channel 4 produced a *National protocol for adoption* (Channel 4, 2000), the key points of which were echoed within a year by the Prime Minister's own review (2001). The social work profession supported all the main proposals in the review, only querying whether sufficient resources would be provided to deliver the agenda. In 2001, the government committed an extra £66.5 million over three years to improve adoption services. It also introduced statutory paternity leave for adoptive fathers in 2000.

As well as these positive moves, there is a consensus about the importance of key professional processes that need to take place for a successful individual adoption and a successful local adoption system, in particular: a robust and regularly reviewed care plan for the child; a thorough assessment of the prospective adopter; a good matching of child with adopter; preparation of the child for placement; good post-placement support; and well-run disruption meetings to try to keep the placement on track or to end it by mutual agreement if it breaks down irretrievably. In addition, regular widespread local and national publicity is required to bring new adopters forward in large numbers.

While it is important not to over-state concerns, the current system is fragile. Confidence in local authority adoption agencies is low, with better performance and better reputation management essential – far too many opinion formers from all walks of life tell stories about how their attempts to adopt were frustrated by mystifying processes and bungled bureaucracy. At the risk of repeating ourselves, another basic problem is the structural shortage of adopters. Trade magazines, like *Children who wait*, published bi-monthly by Adoption Today, and *Be my parent*, published by BAAF Adoption and Fostering, also bi-monthly, are packed out with the profiles of children needing adopters, for whom insufficient people have come forward to date. Sophisticated fertility treatments and assisted conception techniques, such as GIFT (Gamete Intra Fallopian Transfer) or ICSI (Intra Cytoplasmic Sperm Injection), may make it easier for childless couples to have their own children rather than adopt, which may in turn further limit the numbers of potential adopters in the future. All adoption agencies agree that an adoption assessment should not be started while people are receiving fertility treatment or are trying to conceive a baby.

One key issue identified by the government is the delay in some parts of the country in placing children who should be adopted. However, the government also freely acknowledges the reasons for delay are varied. They include the extensive preparation some children need before they can be adopted, if a high risk of placement breakdown is to be avoided; delays in police checks on prospective adopters, sometimes for months; shortages of social workers, which are chronic in some parts of the UK and which lead in turn to low morale amongst remaining staff; and delays in the legal process, including scheduling difficulties, which necessitate active judicial management of each set of adoption proceedings.

New specialist court centres, which started in late 2001, should help reduce delays through cases being handled by specialist adoption judges and court adoption officers. The tension between the political executive and the judiciary remains however, and there are warning signs from the United States about what happens when policy makers act in isolation. Federal law requires states to seek termination of parental rights for almost any child in foster care for 15 of the most recent 22 months. Yet in many jurisdictions, it can take at least 12 months for a judge to decide if the initial placement was justified in the first place. 'And this influx of new termination cases comes despite increasing evidence that the system can't cope with the thousands of children legally free for adoption right now' (National Coalition for Child Protection Reform, 2000). The judiciary itself, perhaps mourning the loss of its old wardship powers, has been considering keeping a small number of cases under review in the courts, using a 'starred care plan' system.

Where there are serious delays, it is often due to rival applications to adopt from relatives or foster carers coming in late, just as cases come to court for a final decision; or a genuine shortage of a suitable adopter for a specific child or, increasingly, a sibling group. Birth parents contest adoptions in nearly 60 per cent of cases, which lengthens the time taken to make a final determination. The natural father of Belinda and Kimberley Kilshaw was the last to register an interest in the 'Internet twins'. Elsewhere in the US, a 20-year-old airline flight attendant challenged his 16-month-old son's adoption on the grounds that he was unaware of the child's existence (*Guardian*, 5 December 2000). Unmarried fathers are a new group who, in pushing their own rights, will, in most cases, make the legal situation more complex to resolve. This will extend the delay for a child before she or he can settle into a new family and make a permanent attachment. Equally, the claims of natural fathers to adopt their own children alone have been validated in the British courts (In *re: B (a minor) Adoption: natural parent*, House of Lords decision, 17 December 2001).

Delay is justified if something essential to the adoption process is happening. Delay cannot be justified if no action is being taken. Delays in the adoption process can occur because either a local authority or a guardian ad litem instructs an expert witness, usually to assess an aspect of an individual child's needs where these are not clear. This can skew the timetable and add months to the court process. In order to meet stiffer government targets, adoption agencies will have to change their ways of working. This will entail their ensuring all children looked after for six months have a permanence plan; using concurrent or parallel planning (see Chapter 3), so that potential adopters are identified early; holding adoption panels more frequently, possibly weekly in larger authorities; employing a specialist solicitor to work as a member of the adoption team, so that delays in the court process can be minimised; and ensuring that applicants are dealt with positively and quickly at every stage of the adoption process.

Some consultancies have produced high quality material to assist local authorities in improving performance. The government's Adoption and Permanence Taskforce is also developing new approaches such as a visual tracking tool to monitor the care pathway of a child from the last care episode to an adoption order, as a means of ensuring that the National Adoption Standards are embedded at the casework level. Adoption agencies have responded to this call. According to the government's own inspectors, the vast majority of councils, who still form the bulk of adoption agencies, are improving their performance, and have given adoption a higher profile (Department of Health, 2001).

The government's policy of adoption at any cost has risks. It may force black children into unsuitable white homes simply because these are more likely to be available and usable within the 12-month time limit for placement. On the other hand, in some parts of the country, there is a shortage of white adopters and a surfeit of black adopters, so generalisations are dangerous. There may be a temptation to try quick fixes or magic solutions, for example to place too many children with one willing adopter. Jeanette Roberts was described as a saint on the BBC *Children in need* programme because she adopted and fostered over thirty-five children. She was also the subject of documentaries and books about positive child care, and she attracted more than £1 million in funding to a charitable trust she had created. But she was described by a judge as a liar and a risk to children, after it was found she subjected several children she looked after to emotional, physical and financial abuse, including encouraging children to make allegations of sexual abuse against their parents.

While the care she offered undoubtedly benefited some children, who felt a lifelong loyalty to her, Roberts was unmanageable as a carer in a series of contractual arrangements with local authorities, although part of her defence was that those local authorities showed little human interest in the children she was looking after. One problem for the authorities in realising what was going on was that each placement with her was handled individually. No one took an overview. The costs of investigations and court costs incurred by Essex County Council amounted to £4.8 million.

A requirement to place children at the speed the government proposes may require greater incentives: higher fees and tax concessions for adopters and maybe a bounty for local authorities such as that paid in the US by the federal government to states, in which states are paid $4,000–$6,000 for every finalised adoption above a baseline number. (Here the government is moving towards this with its public service agreements and Performance Fund targets agreed with local authorities but not voluntary adoption agencies.) A third incentive could be a new national adoption support service, available around the clock for adopters to consult if they need help or advice.

The shortfall in the numbers of people approved for adoption also applies to foster carers. Indeed, many foster carers adopt a child or children originally placed with them as a short-term placement, so that even though converting such placements into adoptive placements is good news for the individual child or children concerned, it means other children cannot benefit from the potential fostering placement and the overall pool of foster carers goes down, unless new carers are recruited. New carers in significant numbers will only be found from currently under-represented groups such as people over 40 and single people. Making less restrictive the conventional criteria to adopt will be a prerequisite of a successful national adoption service in the future. A study carried out for BAAF Adoption and Fostering by MORI found that the general public would support such a move. Sixty-eight per cent of people agreed that unmarried couples in stable long-term relationships should be eligible to adopt jointly, with only 18 per cent disagreeing (BAAF Adoption and Fostering, 2001).

Potential adopters want an efficient follow up to their initial enquiry; a choice of adoption agencies; independent advice; a sharing of information; life story books; training; different support at different times; and immediate access to effective help in a crisis (Adoption UK, 2000). Adoption UK, a network of adopter support groups, formed in 1971, has developed a compre-hensive training programme for adopters called *It's a piece of cake*. Using songs, child profiles, fictional characters, feelings lists, spidograms, and all manner of interesting and stimulating material assembled as stand-alone but linked modules, *It's a piece of cake* illustrates a growing sophistication in resource material on adoption.

Adoption, like infertility treatment, and medically produced designer babies, give new options for would-be parents. Modern motherhood is a technological frontier, so it is hardly surprising that trends in adoption, like Internet adoption, also move with the times. The definition of a family is being constantly revised. What is most interesting and curious is that in this age of reconstituted families, serial relationships, same sex marriages, and the preference of many people to remain single, at least until well into their thirties, 95 per cent of adoptions involve stable married heterosexual couples, contrary to the myth that politically correct social workers will do all they can to avoid such placements. The reality of adoption is seen through a series of distorting mirrors. The alarm expressed by a husband 30 years ago when his wife decided she wanted to adopt, is also not uncommon today. The couple had been married for 10 years and had not been able to have a family. 'I feel this [adoption] would be an insult to my manhood . . . I wonder if you can realise how important it is for a man to be a real father' (*Scottish Daily Express*, 11 May 1972). Adoption work defies simplistic generalisation.

Another core concern is that children's services in the UK, including adoption services, remain severely under-resourced. It is estimated that just less than half a million children in the UK can be catergorised as children in need. The main task for a limited number of child care staff, in teams often carrying high levels of vacancies due to long-term recruitment problems, is to prevent children needing to go into state care in the first place. Putting disproportionate resources into family placement services runs the same risks as that run by the health service when it starves primary care of resources and pours resources into hospitals and acute care. Local authorities already put more than 50 per cent of their total child care budgets into looked-after children. Even more worrying is the increasing percentage of family placement budgets going to independent fostering agencies, who charge up to double the cost of local authority placements.

The need to properly resource prevention services is heightened as the rate of family breakdown in the UK is increasing, as are births outside marriage. The increase in lone parents in the UK means that a similar increase in local family support services is essential. The widening gap between rich and poor in the UK is also a key factor. It is estimated that about 22 per cent of children in the UK are living in families where the income is half that of the average wage (NCH Action for Children, 2000). The number of temporary homeless households is also increasing. More children with complex disabilities are surviving because of improved neo-natal care and they are another group needing more and better support services in the home.

Black children have been over-represented in the care system for 50 years and social policy has scarcely budged – a breath-taking continuity. Campaigns like the Soulkids campaign in the late 1970s and Rowe and Lambert's research (1973) at the same time which showed that while white children were being placed in families, black children were more often than not left stranded in residential care, first focused attention on the scale of the problem. The same imbalance remains today, especially for children with a mixed parentage requiring a placement. Research by Ince (1988) shows that 26 per cent of black children in care are waiting for a family.

Some commentators are convinced racism is alive and well and still undermining the welfare of black children. The views expressed by Josephine Kwhali, head of children and families services, London Borough of Hackney, could have been said 30 years ago when attention was first being drawn to the plight of black children in care. 'Racism and the institutional and personal behaviours which maintain it are internalised by black children and affect their self identity and self esteem. Black children generally, and black boys in particular, are racially pathologised and labelled which affects the recruitment of foster and adoptive carers' (speech at a BAAF Adoption and Fostering seminar, 11 March 2001). Many transracially adopted adults look back on their placements as a form of kidnap. They feel displaced from their native community or community of origin. Some, like Mae Ahmin, an African Caribbean poet transracially placed in Germany and who took her own life in 2000, never recover or grow to feel at home anywhere. While there are many positive and innovative projects like the Khandan initiative run by Barnardo's in Scotland, which seeks to place black children in care in Scotland with same-race carers, such initiatives have by no means become part of the mainstream throughout the UK.

The new National Adoption Standards will help, as will the Race Relations (Amendment) Act, 2001, both of which strengthen the requirement on public bodies to deliver on the equalities agenda. Within those standards, care needs to be taken not to discriminate unwittingly against carers from ethnic minority communities. For example, if the same standards for room sizes were used for children's bedrooms in foster homes as are used in residential care homes for adults, 75 per cent of Asian applicants to foster in Bradford would be excluded. Similarly, in some case conferences, the first language should often be non-English, with an interpreter being used to translate meetings not English for English speakers present. Some inner city information leaflets for adoption positively reflect diversity. Islington's has pictures and quotations from two mixed race adopters (a black woman and a white man in one; a white woman and a black man in another); a gay male couple; a single parent; and a black adoptive couple. They may have gone too far as the only adopters not represented in the literature are white couples.

The pace of change in the adoption world is quickening. The Adoption and Children Act 2002 is set to introduce a raft of changes to the UK adoption system, the most significant of which are:

• Giving prospective adopters the right to a fully independent review of their case if they are turned down by an adoption panel.

- Giving adopters a right to an assessment by their council for post-placement support and a legal power or duty to provide support for as long as it is needed or when a need specifically arises.
- Establishing a new 'special guardianship' option for children, which does not sever the legal tie with birth parents.
- Requiring councils to pay the court fees when looked-after children are adopted (at the moment, some councils do and some don't).
- Stipulating that local authorities should increase the number of their children looked after who are adopted by half by 2004–5.
- Establishing an adoption register for England and Wales (to be expanded to Scotland and Northern Ireland at a later date) both for children waiting more than six months to be adopted and for families approved for adoption.
- Reducing delays by increasing the number of judges able to do family work and to train more court officials (there are a number of examples where court staff have sent the details of adoptive parents directly to birth parents).
- Updating adoption legislation by aligning the Adoption Act 1976 with the Children Act 1989.
- Ensuring that when adoption is right for a child in care, that the decision to place for adoption is made within six months and that a family is found within a further six months (so that the adoption process lasts a similar length for a parent to the length of natural childbirth).
- Relaxing the rules on unmarried couples being able to adopt.

Several key issues remain though, some of them not yet addressed. They include:

- Whether a national adoption agency outside local authorities would fundamentally transform the shortcomings of the current system. However popular this might be, the experience to date of Whitehall-administered services like the Children and Family Court Advisory and Support Service is not encouraging.
- Updating adoption legislation by aligning the Adoption Act 1976 with the Children Act 1989, for example by ensuring that placement orders simplify the adoption process by securing a child in a particular placement; or allowing removal from it, in the period before a full adoption order is made or considered.
- Whether to standardise adoption allowances nationally, and allow them to be claimed after an adoption order is made as well as before, in cases where an adoptive family's financial circumstances worsen years into adoption.
- Redefining the relevance of religious background in adoptions, as religious practice changes dramatically in the UK, from a decreasing emphasis in some communities to assuming an ever-greater significance in others. Race and culture also need to be redefined, as complex mixed

parentage becomes more common, and harder to match when finding an adoptive family.

For government policy to be successful, the many groups involved in the adoption process have to believe in it. The only groups who wholeheartedly support the new push for adoption are the government and adopters. Most people with a stake in the adoption system accept that many individual children wait a disgracefully long period in care, sometimes to the point where they become unadoptable. On the other hand, few want to see adoption elevated over and above other child care solutions like family support and kinship care. Too much emphasis on adoption goes hand in hand with under-recognition of other equally important areas of childcare practice, which have good success rates if resources and expertise are committed to them. Adoption is a political football and could become an own goal for its advocates without a sense of proportion and perspective (Douglas, 2001).

Let us end with a story that illustrates the whole purpose of this book – to reveal the changing face of adoption today. Heather, a birth mother, placed a message on the internet site, 'Missing You', asking for the son whom she gave up for adoption to contact her. A year later she received a telephone call from his wife. Heather rang her son, Colin, and, after 35 years, they arranged to meet. Two years later they remain in contact by telephone, email and text message. She is 54 and he is 37. Colin wanted to trace his birth father and Heather found him – living on a catamaran in New Zealand. They plan to travel together to the other side of the world to meet him. All the partners and the children in the linked families are delighted and thrilled at acquiring new relatives – another sign of our times.

In a world increasingly characterised as a global village, this story shows that, the end of past legal barriers aside, there are now new opportunities for reunion. But it also shows that happy endings are not just possible – they are being fought for and achieved.

References

Adoption UK (2000), *An adopter's perspective*, Banbury, Adoption UK.

BAAF Adoption and Fostering (2001), *Attitudes to adoption: summary findings* (research study), London, BAAF Adoption and Fostering.

Channel 4 (2000), *National protocol on adoption*, London, Channel 4 Publications.

Department of Health (2000), *Adopting changes*, London, Department of Health.

Douglas, A. (2001), Viewpoints on adoption, *The Magistrate*, January.

Ince, L. (1988), *Making it alone. A study of the care experiences of black people*, London, British Agencies for Adoption and Fostering.

National Coalition for Child Protection Reform (2000), *Family preservation and adoption*, Issue paper 13, Virginia, US.

NCH Action for Children (2000), *Factfile 1999: facts and figures on issues facing Britain's children*, London, NCH Action for Children.

Rowe, J. and Lambert, L. (1973), *Children who wait*, London, Association of Agencies for Adoption and Fostering.

27

HOME NEWS AND ABROAD

Comparing UK trends elsewhere

June Thoburn

Central to this chapter on the likely future of adoption is an awareness that the 'closed' 'fresh start' model of adoption, still dominant in much western thinking, is essentially Eurocentric and of very short duration in the total history of the informal and formal adoptive family. It will start by considering the global context of the future of adoption for the key stakeholders: birth parents and relatives; children; families considering adoption; and agencies responsible for securing the welfare of children in need. Since the passing of the Adoption Act 1926 (the basic philosophical stance of which has not been substantially altered by subsequent UK legislation) the world has become more intimately connected. From the Oedipus myth and the story of Moses, adoption has always been, at least in part, about children as a commodity, bringing potential benefit to the adoptive family; and as a threat to the personal safety or future prosperity and wellbeing of the birth family. In a minority of cases it has been about greed (selling a child to the highest bidder) exploitation and victimisation of children through domestic slavery or pornography. Last, and happily in the majority of cases, it has been about altruism, whether that means giving up a child to save his or her life or ensure a better life, or taking into one's home a child needing special care and commitment.

In the second half of the twentieth century, improved transport and communications have meant that adoption has moved from something that happens between families or within communities to something which can occur across continents. With the reduction in fertility rates in families in the developed world, coupled with the reduced availability of babies for adoption within their home communities, children have become an international commodity. These trends have led to the implementation of human rights legislation and international conventions (most notably the UN Convention on the Rights of the Child and the Hague Convention on Adoption) in an attempt to protect the interests not only of the children but also of their birth relatives, often children themselves, who are usually the most vulnerable members of their societies. Within these conventions there is scope for the size of privately organised adoption to vary, provided that the child's rights and welfare are safeguarded. In summary, all children have the right to be protected from maltreatment and to grow up in their own families or the countries and culture in which they were born. Only when their welfare and protection needs cannot be met in their home environments should the state step in to secure the severance of legal ties with the birth family (or country of birth) and legally to join the child to a new family by adoption. However, the private market in adoptable children flourishes more in some countries (especially in US 'in-country' adoptions and in some Central and South American 'sending countries'). This global context has to be the starting point for a consideration of the future of adoption in the UK, because UK governments cannot control the impact of global trends in adoption; at best they can only regulate them. On the positive side, globalisation, international conventions and better communications provide the opportunity for legislators and child welfare agencies to look at the ways in which other countries seek to meet the needs of children for whom adoption may be appropriate. In the past, the UK has looked more across the Atlantic than across the North Sea for inspiration, but recent human rights legislation may sit more happily with a European perspective.

What, then, is the likely future of adoption in the UK? As earlier chapters have shown, UK adoption policy and practice have some similarities but many differences with practice in all other countries. We share with other developed countries a situation in which the choice of adoption as a response to an unplanned pregnancy has greatly diminished. In England and Wales, around 200 newborn babies are currently placed for adoption each year at the request of their parents (down from around 8,500 in 1970). The fall is even more striking in other European countries. The testimony of birth parents (some writing in this volume) suggests that they are probably right to avoid the (still unquantified) risk of long-term trauma resulting from such a major separation and loss, now that welfare systems and changed social attitudes make it unnecessary to face the alternative of a life of poverty and stigma. In the US, universalist welfare services are less adequate and recent legislation in some states has indeed cut further the right to welfare payments and health care. Thus the number of infants placed 'voluntarily' for adoption through state and voluntary agencies, and by private arrangements, remains comparatively high. In the developing world and transitional economies of central Europe, absolute poverty, high rates of parent mortality, the costs of health care and education for older children still drive families to abandon their babies, or give them up to state care and consent to adoption mainly by childless couples from overseas.

Developing countries share with those in the developed world the experience of increasing social fragmentation and problems of family violence, mental illness, criminality and addictions which require state intervention to protect the well-being of children. The cushion of universal health and income maintenance systems and family support services keeps the numbers actually coming into state care lower in Europe, Australasia and Canada than in the US. Nevertheless, they all share the task of finding ways to provide for the long-term well-being of increasing numbers of children who cannot be brought up safely by their birth parents, and in all countries most of these children are older, have disabilities or show in their behaviour the scars of early maltreatment or neglect. The emphasis in all countries is to keep as many of these children as possible within the extended family or community. Differences emerge when we look at the use of adoption as a route to permanence for children in care. The Performance and Innovations Unit (PIU, 2000) reports that of 11 countries profiled, only the UK and the US place substantial numbers from care for adoption. The marked difference with other European countries is explained by differing views about whether it is ethically and legally possible to place children for adoption when birth parents do not consent. A substantial part of the difference between the US and the UK rates of placement from care for adoption is explained by the fact that adoption by relatives accounts for around 14 per cent of US adoptions from care and is considered either unnecessary or undesirable in the UK, and that almost half are by short-term foster parents with whom the child is already living (PIU, 2000, p. 81). This trend (around 30 per cent in 1999) is growing in the UK, but the majority of adoptions are still by people not previously known to the child.

Is the pattern for the future already written into the script, or are changes to be anticipated? What can research and recent history tell us about what the future might hold for the 'adoption prism' – the birth families, adoptees, adopters and agencies?

As has already been noted, very few pregnant women in the UK now look to adoption as the solution to unplanned pregnancy and there is little to suggest that this will change. If anything, the numbers will go down even further. At the moment, though numerically small, a larger than expected proportion of infants placed voluntarily for adoption have one or both parents of South Asian ethnic origin (Neil, 2000). The explanation is likely to lie in the stigma and isolation from the community likely to be faced by a young Asian woman who has a baby outside marriage. It may well be that, like their English counterparts in the 1970s and Irish Catholic young women in the 1990s, they will reject the community's sanctions and decide not to give up their babies. From time to time a politician or other public figure calls on more young women to be persuaded to give up their babies for adoption. There is no sign that this is happening, nor is there any evidence that social workers or other professionals persuade young women to keep their babies. There is some suggestion that peer-group pressure comes down against adoption but what seems more likely is that birth families rally around and young mothers, and sometimes fathers, decide for themselves that they have the capacity to bring up their children. On the other hand, global poverty seems likely to ensure a steady stream of babies and young children from poor countries being adopted by those in the developed world who have the financial resources and determination to succeed. The countries from which these children come will change as some shrug off the worst ravages of poverty. For example, China, a major 'sender' country now, is developing and formalising its services for domestic adoption. African families and communities, arguably most in need of adoption services for the many AIDS orphans, show no sign of seeing large scale adoption overseas as part of a solution to the very large numbers who would fit the UN Convention definition of children in need for whom adoption outside their home communities might be appropriate. The flow from South America and Russia shows no sign of stopping and, as the case of the 'Internet twins' and the Kilshaws reminded us, poor families in the US see adoption of their children, sometimes overseas, as a way out of poverty.

Evidence from the US, Australia and New Zealand, where birth parents have a stronger say in the adoption of their children, suggests that British birth parents who do choose adoption (often having originally rejected the idea but finding themselves no longer able to cope) will join many of those whose children are adopted from care against their consent in asking for their children to be placed with adopters who will facilitate continuing birth family contact. This trend is likely to increase with the changes in adoption law which strengthen the requirement for birth parents to be provided with a service in their own right. With the help of advocates able to put their case, and the human rights legislation and the 'right to family life' in the background, it may be less easy for their wishes about continuing contact to be over-ruled. This may also mean that more children in care are placed with permanent foster families or under the terms of a special guardianship order. The growing use of family group conferences to aid decisions about permanence options may also lead to more placements of children in care with relatives, for whom special guardianship rather than adoption is likely to be most appropriate.

It seems likely that the numbers of UK-born infants needing adoptive families will remain low. The majority of those in the youngest group will have been removed from their parents at birth, presenting a special challenge to the adopters to empathise with and help the child to understand a story far removed from the traditional adoption story. 'You are living in this family because your mother killed your brother before you were born' is a far cry from 'your mum wanted you to have a mummy and a daddy and to carry on with her schooling'. Most will be placed from care having already experienced neglect or maltreatment and a smaller number will be placed because they have severe disabilities with which their birth parents feel unable to cope. UK social workers have a proud record of placing children from care with permanent substitute families, sometimes for adoption and sometimes as foster children and UK families can be proud of their record of taking into their homes children of all ages with some very severe physical and emotional problems (see Fratter *et al.*, 1991, Thoburn, 1999, Lowe *et al.*, 1999 for summaries of the development of permanence policies for looked-after children in the UK).

The research is clear that some individual children are 'unadoptable', either because they do not wish to be adopted or have been so damaged by earlier experiences that the risk to the new family and the risk of harm to the child from another failed experience of family life would be too high. An average breakdown rate of 20 per cent for children placed from care with families not previously known to them has brought home the message that finding the family and placing the child is only the first step along a potentially bumpy road to a successful placement. However the research is also clear that no group of children is un-adoptable, whether defined by age, ethnicity, disability, needing to be placed with siblings, or needing to preserve links with the birth family. There has been a trend in the last few years for the proportion of children placed when under the age of four to increase, and the actual numbers and proportions of school age children to decrease. There is a risk that league tables, added to the rigid application to older children of time limits framed around the needs of infants and toddlers, will accelerate this trend. It may be that long-term foster care and special guardianship are more appropriate options for older children but for some, including some teenagers, adoption is the right choice. Adoption of a teenager has the same chance of success as for a nine- or ten-year-old if he or she is committed to finding a new family and care is taken with the matching process and post-placement support. On the other hand, pressure to place older children within rigidly interpreted time scales could increase breakdown rates if children are placed before they are ready or with families who are unable to meet important identified needs.

For some years now, adoption of a 'straightforward' relinquished infant has ceased to be a way forward for all but a tiny minority of the involuntary childless. For them, there is more hope in advances in assisted reproduction, though some will continue to look to overseas adoption. The essential characteristics of the successful adoptive family of the future are already well known. The major question is, can the resources be made available to encourage them to come forward, complete home studies and support them in the numbers needed even to reach the present target for England of placing 5,000 children from care each year? Or, more fundamentally, do they exist in the numbers needed? Indicators of likely success are not to be found in demographic characteristics such as age, marital status, childlessness or experienced parents, or in characteristics such as sexual orientation or any particular motivation. Those recruiting adopters will be looking for less measurable attributes such as flexibility, determination, enjoying a challenge, and the ability to see success in small steps forward. Since some form of continuing contact with birth family members will be a part of most adoptions, the ability to empathise not only with the child but also with the child's (often distressing) history, and with the birth parents themselves, will be much in demand as a characteristic for the successful adopter of the future. Given the many problems the children face, an element of post-placement support and the involvement (at least episodically) with social workers and other helping professionals is likely to be part of adoptive family life.

There is little sign so far of UK adoption agencies following their counterparts in the US and the rest of Europe in devoting more of their energies to inter-country adoption. If they were to do so in the near future at a time when the shortage of qualified social workers is acute, this could only be at the expense of children in care in the UK who need adoptive families. An alternative might be for the Department for International Development, in the spirit of the Hague Convention, to view international adoption for children for whom there is no alternative as a form of overseas aid. They would then make adequate funds available and fund social work nationals in the 'sender' countries to undertake the work with birth parents and children. Crystal ball gazing is slightly easier with the passing of the Adoption and Children Act. This was largely welcomed by those voluntary and local authority adoption agencies whose progressive work with all parts of the 'adoption circle' finds support in the detailed proposals, especially for post-adoption services. The Act makes it clear that if adoption is to remain a route out of care for all those children for whom it is appropriate, it must remain firmly embedded within the services for looked-after children. Successful adoption work starts with high quality practice with birth parents and children before entry to care, and when the care plan is being arrived at. Building a picture of the child's needs and the wishes and potential for future involvement in the placement process of the birth parents relatives and siblings is essential for successful matching. If the matching process fails to meet the child's needs, even high quality post-placement work will, at best, be papering over the cracks.

A review of the permanent family placement outcome research from around the world suggests that once placed, whether with adoptive families, foster families or through legal guardianship, the majority of placements made with the intention that they will provide the child with a family for life succeed in meeting most of the children's needs and bring fulfilment and a sense of satisfaction to most of the new parents. However, a disruption rate of around one in five for children placed from care when past infancy must remain a cause for concern. The provisions in the new legislation for avoiding unnecessary delay, broadening the range of legal options, and providing post-adoption support services to children, adopters and birth parents have the potential to increase the numbers placed and improve the success rates. However, the challenges are many and improvements will not be achieved unless adequate funding and social work time are invested in all aspects of the service.

References

Fratter, J., Rowe, J., Sapsford, D. and Thoburn, J. (1991), *Permanent family placement: a decade of experience*, London, British Agencies for Adoption and Fostering.

Lowe, N., Murch, M., Borkowski, M., Weaver, A., Beckford, V. and Thomas, C. (1999), *Supporting adoption*, London, British Agencies for Adoption and Fostering.

Neil, E. (2000), The reasons why young children are placed for adoption: findings from a recently placed sample and a discussion of implications for future identity issues, *Child and Family Social Work*, 4(6), 303–16.

Performance and Innovation Unit (2000), *Review of adoption: issues for consultation*, London, Cabinet Office.

Thoburn, J. (1999), Trends in foster care and adoption, in O. Stevenson (ed.), *Child welfare in the UK*, Oxford, Blackwell Science.

28

ADOPTION SERVICES IN LOCAL AUTHORITIES

Penny Thompson and Nick Hughes

In less than a decade, adoption has moved from being a small specialist subject, the province of a few experienced workers with little interest shown by senior managers, to being a service at the heart of children and families services, and one of the key areas of public interest and government monitoring.

The reasons for this heightened focus are fourfold. First, adoption has caught the imagination of the media, because a number of influential people have been able to draw attention to it and to question the professionalism of social workers who are said to be over bureaucratic, politically correct and a law unto themselves.

Second, with the advent of a more strategic approach to the provision of services to children and families in need, family placements and adoption specifically have become part of the continuum of provision for children looked after. Adoption provides a permanent option for a small group of children looked after, about whom there has been increasing public concern, and hence increasing interest in how best to help.

Third, research into evidence about what works for children who have experienced early childhood disruption and damage, has given encouragement to managers and practitioners to seek permanent substitute care for those children who cannot remain with their birth family. Adoption is foremost amongst the preferred options for permanent family placements, especially for younger children.

Fourth, the contraction of residential care has given a renewed profile to family placements. For the majority of children looked after, this is a temporary state and they return to their family of origin or kinship network. However, for a small number of children, permanent substitute parenting is required and adoption is often the permanent solution of choice, both for the child and for substitute families, whereas children would have languished in long-term residential care until relatively recently.

233

Of 700 children looked after in Sheffield, about 60–75 children require adoption (2001). A similar number need a permanent fostering placement or perhaps with the advent of new legislation, a special guardianship order. They are generally children with profound needs for whom placements are not easy to find. The numbers may be small, but their needs are great.

In modern practice then, what is in it for the adopter? An often demanding and damaged child, possibly tricky contact arrangements, and a media ready to pounce if things go wrong. Apart from councils, the rest of the public sector including health and education agencies are not signed up nationally to taking a full role and making a real financial commitment to children looked after. In addition, we have under-resourced, under-staffed and under-skilled children's services which are frantically trying to juggle a raft of equally competing demands.

To answer these real dilemmas, central government and social services are forging a partnership by devising standards, drafting legislation and jointly staffing a taskforce. The taskforce is bringing together high achieving authorities with those who need to make progress, in order to transfer learning and provide support to service improvement strategies.

The government is determined to increase the number of children benefiting from a permanent family life. For social services departments, this policy direction is welcome, and is being responded to with vigour, supported by the Quality Protects grant regime. Good practice is characterised by:

- A dedicated skilled team to recruit and train potential adopters, backed up by other specialist child care teams like a children with disabilities team.
- An explicit training and recruitment strategy.
- Genuine inter-agency working.
- A regional or sub-regional approach to share knowledge, recruitment skills and best practice.
- A regional or sub-regional core training programme to ensure common standards, enable smaller authorities to bring down waiting times for applicants who can attend a course elsewhere, and enable fast tracking in larger ones.
- Conducting and implementing best value reviews.
- Building in robust and real links between managers of children looked after teams, and family placement teams, in order to promote skills, share knowledge and iron out issues in a practical way.
- Ensuring permanent fostering and residency options have their right place, neither as a poor relation nor as a bad compromise.

Government interest in, and action on adoption indicates national recognition for the enduring place of adoption in children's services. But adoption has to change fundamentally and must be recognised as a legal state requiring both financial and professional support. The advent of the National Adoption Register will assist in increasing the availability of adoptive placements, but only by increasing the numbers of potential adopters will we enable those children who can be adopted to be placed within a reasonable timescale, while at the same time meeting their cultural and religious needs. And to increase the number of children who are adopted we must have more applicants.

To attract more adopters, we have to improve the image and understanding of adoption and improve responsiveness to enquiries. To this end, recruitment and assessment practice must be designed to respond swiftly and effectively to interested potential adopters, and to make sound matching recommendations to adoption panels. The skills of marketing and service promotion are now key to effective adoption agencies, as well as the more traditional assessment and decision-making skills.

Happily, adoption is one of the areas identified for the next round of applications for Beacon status, thus giving a chance to highlight success and offer evidence of what works in local authorities nationally.

Post-adoption services began slowly following the Children Act 1989. This area of multi-agency work must develop at a pace to ensure the provision of an effective child-centred adoption service. The taskforce will take the chance to highlight and promote those authorities and agencies in the vanguard of post-adoption practice.

Not only do local authorities need to develop adoption as part of a comprehensive service, and to have effective recruitment and assessment practice and post-adoption support for children. They also need to improve their development of effective practice in the preparation of children for long-term and permanent placements.

In recent years, increasing emphasis has been given to the importance of initial assessments to safeguard children, identify risks and to plan for their longer-term future. The Department of Health Assessment Framework, linking as it does to the Looked After Children Materials, has helped to raise standards. Training in assessment and decision making continues to be at the heart of children's services employee development plans. There is no more important decision than that which places a child in permanent substitute care. The need for sound permanency planning and decision making is critical.

It may well be that there should be a review of performance indicators to ensure they can gauge the quality of permanence planning and the work being undertaken, once such a plan has been determined.

Following a decision for a permanent alternative placement, there is a need for effective direct work with children to prepare them for placement. There is a challenge to social services to develop, value and resource direct work with children, and the Department of Health to disseminate evidence-based knowledge about the preparation of children for placement. There is an opportunity here for guidance to support the new adoption standards. The importance of preparation, which addresses key issues including loss, separation and capacity to move on, is critical to the future well-being of the individual child as evidenced by research on long-term outcomes.

In recent years the concept of corporate parenting has been developed in local authorities to describe the responsibility across the whole local authority, including housing, education and leisure, for looked-after children, recognising that social services cannot meet all corporate parent responsibilities without the active involvement of the rest of the local authority.

With the development of modern adoption focusing as it does on a wide age range and a demanding set of needs, the powers described in the Children Act 1989 have become duties under the Adoption and Children Act 2002 for the provision of post-adoption support. No longer does the adoption order signal the end of local authority involvement with the child and its new family. Rather, many children who are adopted will require support and assistance in the years following their adoption, while help from health, education or social services will be essential. The question for local authorities is whether they can, in partnership with health and other organisations, give attention and help to children when they have been adopted, whilst avoiding negative labelling or stigmatising these children as no longer having a legitimate claim on services or resources.

Moreover, a really effective post-adoption support service has resource implications. Nationally, children's services within social services are struggling to meet increasing need and rising expectations within allocated resources. Further service development cannot be achieved without additional resources and without it becoming a priority for other agencies. Children's services will benefit from a new National Service Framework from 2003, which is likely to make the involvement of other agencies mandatory.

Of equal importance are considerations like shortages of staff; training and development needs; workload management; and, as indicated above, the need to address a shortage of adopters. The new national demands will take time to meet, and many factors militate against it.

Adoption should be central to any professionally sound children and families service in a local authority. For small authorities, it may well be that the assessment and provision of adopters is transferred to a voluntary agency or to a consortium. In those authorities, the focus will be on assessment and planning. In larger authorities, capacity has to be created to fulfil the varied aspects of assessment planning and the provision of sufficient resources. This is too often at the expense of other services which are not as critical but which nevertheless matter just as much to local people.

For all authorities large or small, there is a need to reinvent adoption as one of a range of permanent options for children, for whom a return to their family of birth is impossible but for whom the chance to grow up in a family is their right. At the same time, public confidence in the service has to increase if we are to attract the volume and range of adopters for the many children who wait for a new chance of a permanent family. The following examples illustrate how few decisions in child care today are straightforward.

Jake is 6½ years old and has a Pakistani (Muslim) father and white (Catholic) mother. He has special educational needs. He shares the same mother with Sue, aged 6 months, who is of wholly white (Catholic) parentage and is developing normally. Jake is very proud and protective of his baby sister. The court has agreed a plan for adoption for both children. Despite blanket advertising and seeking help through BAAF Fostering and Adoption link there has been no interest in Jake.

There are any number of approved adopters ready and willing to take Sue. Some are practising Catholics. Sue and Jake are in the same foster placement. These carers, who are lapsed Anglicans, would be happy to keep Sue but are not keen to have Jake. However, they say if the price of keeping Sue, who is a really pretty baby, is having Jake too, then so be it. 'She's worth it', they say. The birth father has been rejected by his family as they are strict practising Muslims and he wants nothing more to do with Jake or social services. As far as his family are concerned, Jake 'does not exist'. The children's birth mother has disappeared but, despite not practising herself, has expressed a wish that Sue be placed with practising Catholics – she has warm memories of going to mass. She does not care what happens to Jake.

Let us now take the sibling group of three who have been placed in a foster family for the last three years. It has not been possible to find an adoptive placement for all three yet. The children are nine, seven, five. The foster carers will adopt the two youngest but not the oldest.

Another case concerns Sheila, a 32-year-old white lone parent, and John, her partner, who is also white. They have been referred because of the concerns around the parenting of Kirsty, their two-year-old daughter, and Tom, her six-year-old half-brother who is a very demanding boy. Tom, who is of mixed race, was returned to Sheila after the breakdown of his placement with extended family on his father's side in another local authority.

Sheila has six other children all by different fathers in different parts of the country, ranging from the eldest who is aged 17, and the subject of a residence order made in favour of her father, to the youngest who is aged four and has been adopted. The other four are either in long-term fostering, or with extended family members, some on court orders, some abandoned there. Every assessment of Sheila has said she has too many needs of her own ever to parent children. Each time she has a child, she and her new partner have demanded to be reassessed as the father has claimed he will provide the necessary support – but they never do. She has said she will go on having children until she is allowed to keep one.

The current problem is the usual pattern. Sheila is unable to cope with the children, and the signs are her relationship with John is coming to an end – they keep breaking up and getting back together. Neither of them want Tom, who they are demanding be accommodated but currently they are back together and claim they will be getting married soon. In the meantime, they fight, argue, drink excessively and their care of the children is very poor. All the other children have no contact with Sheila but varying degrees of contact with each other.

Then there is the story of three-year-old Ben who was admitted to care with his two older half-siblings, following a history of neglect by his mother. The plan for the older two children was rehabilitation to father, who denied paternity of Ben; therefore, Ben couldn't remain with his half-siblings. The children lived together in the past. The plan for Ben was agreed as adoption. The key issues became separating the children; and post-adoption contact. The older children still see their mother. There is a risk of her discovering the whereabouts of Ben's adopters. Direct contact is agreed but drifts after social workers handed this over to father. Eventually contact stops – there is no contact for 18 months. Further down the line, half-siblings request renewed contact with Ben.

Last, we consider the case of Jay, aged one who was admitted to care following serious child abuse with multiple fractures. Both parents blamed each other. Jay is of mixed race and was placed with maternal grandparents who are white. Following unsupervised contact, Jay is injured again and there are concerns about the grandparents' ability to protect. Jay is removed to foster carers. Adoption becomes the agreed plan.

The key issues are several. Other family members come forward – two aunts from each side of the family, one white and one black. Maternal grandparents request the return of Jay to their care. There is the task of balancing Jay's cultural needs versus safety issues. Jay has attachment to his grandparents and this has implications for future contact if he is placed with his father's side of the family who his maternal grandparents don't get on with. Eventually Jay was placed with a paternal aunt but later mother is 'cleared' of injuring him and requested contact with Jay who by this time is very settled.

These everyday examples of social work practice illustrate the complexity of decision-making in adoption, which is a far cry from the public image of a simple matching process between willing adopters and children who just need a good loving home. Because of the need to change and evolve the way we do things, Sheffield Council commissioned an independent Best Value review of our family placement services and we have followed this up by implementing the key findings. These were:

- Creating a recruitment team to carry out all recruitment and training of foster carers and adopters.
- Establishing a permanence team to cover both fostering and adoption – which has set up a duty line for a rapid response to carers with concerns after placement.
- Establishing teams for looked-after children that cover the city.

- Having monthly meetings between family placement managers and of services for looked-after children.
- The family placement manager to lead on a target for secure attachments for looked-after children in Sheffield.

We have also taken some regional approaches, such as:

- Establishing an adoption consortium, which has helped to place children within the region when they cannot be placed with their own local authority boundaries.
- Meeting five adjoining authorities to share best practice, develop regional recruitment and are currently working to develop a core training for carers programme.
- Under the auspices of the Social Services Inspectorate, we are meeting as a Trent regional family placement group with colleagues from residential care services to define and develop a regional approach to internal and external targets, especially placement choice.

Family placement services in Sheffield, as elsewhere, are under great pressure, but having clear strategies in place can help to raise standards, improve morale, and respond to expectations.

29

A SPECIAL FOCUS

The views from the voluntary sector

Terry Connor

In few other spheres of childcare have voluntary agencies been as influential as in the field of adoption. A combination of agency longevity, innovation in practice and research dissemination has contributed to an authority which is disproportionate to their statistical representation in contemporary adoption.

Speculation about the role of voluntary agencies in adoption tends to surface with the advent of new legislation. Perhaps this is not surprising because all adoption work in the UK started with the voluntary adoption societies, a number of whom had been responsible for de facto adoptions as part of their wider children's work well before the first Adoption Act in 1926 for England and Wales. During the 1950s and 1960s, when moral welfare was a branch of social work, the role of the largely church-based voluntary societies was circumscribed by the climate of an era in which, as one commentator has noted, 'for so many years, chastity outside marriage was virtually government policy and adoption the public face of a deeply private and shameful sin' (Wigmore, 1996). When adoption statistics peaked in 1968, 15 out of every 1,000 babies born had been adopted before they reached their first birthday (Howe *et al.*, 1992). The legacy of these thousands of placements has informed much present day adoption policy and practice. Pioneering work by these same societies with adult adoptees and birth parents has highlighted the fact that, as one visionary had forewarned, authentic facts about unmarried mothers were as scarce then as unproven theories were numerous (Rowe, 1966).

The major sea changes which arrived with the Children Act 1975, which gave local authorities responsibility for a comprehensive adoption service, led to uncertainty in people's minds about the role assigned to the adoption societies. Indeed, an editorial in the journal of the Association of British Adoption and Fostering Agencies suggested that the most difficult task the voluntary adoption societies had to face in their half century of existence was that of mere survival (Association of British Adoption and Fostering Agencies, 1976). This, despite government reassurance that a partnership was envisaged between local authorities and adoption societies on the basis of complementary services without unnecessary duplication which offered an element of choice to birth parents and prospective adopters. The forthcoming Adoption and Children Act 2002 reinforces this message with its statement that 'the facilities of the [adoption] service must be provided in conjunction . . . with registered adoption societies in their area, so that help may be given in a coordinated manner without duplication, omission or avoidable delay'.

Much has changed, however, during the intervening years in the nature of adoption policy and practice, relationships between agencies, and the organisational environment in which they operate. The placement of older children with special needs and learning disabilities, pioneered in this country by Parents For Children, a specialist adoption society established in the 1970s, now forms the bulk of adoption work (see Irving, Chapter 1). Post-adoption work, also pioneered by the voluntary sector as part of their mainstream services or in specialist post-adoption centres, is increasingly recognised as a necessity rather than a luxury for children and families involved in adoption. The principle of central or local government grant aid for the general purposes of voluntary adoption agencies, which offered flexibility in the use of funds and the disappearance of which led to some agency closures, has given way to a new regime of fees, contracts and service level agreements. The more recent advent of unitary authorities has had a further impact on relationships between the sectors and the surviving voluntary adoption societies have now adapted to a very different landscape.

In discussing the role of contemporary voluntary adoption societies, it is important to recognise that the organisations are not homogeneous. They may have common roots in public policy and legislation but they will also have their own cultural history, structure, distinctive organisational features and special characteristics. The balance of their activities may vary in emphasis between direct service provision, facilitating and coordinating policy development, advising and influencing others, campaigning to change attitudes and laws, encouraging self-help and providing mutual support, research and consultancy or indeed a combination of any of these strands. Yet despite its heterogeneity, the voluntary sector can point to certain characteristics which are different from other sectors. Discussion about their future role in adoption must necessarily take into account these fundamental differences because it is the interaction between the common themes which permeate the voluntary sector such as value systems, governance, funding and accountability to multiple stakeholders, on which voluntary agency change and survival will ultimately depend (Billis and Harris, 1996).

The ability to manage change whilst remaining singularly focused, the capacity to produce innovative small scale practice models which can be replicated on a larger scale elsewhere and the facility of getting very different individuals to own common organisational goals are features which have helped shape adoption policy and practice. Within the sector there is a vast body of knowledge and expertise about childcare and adoption drawn from many years of agency experience. This is not to say that similar repositories of experience do not exist in the public sector but, as commentators have noted, staff in voluntary adoption agencies are generally more specialised in the sense that they are more likely to devote most or all of their time to adoption work. Those interviewed in the Pathways study had usually spent more than three-quarters of their time on activities directly connected with adoption (Lowe et al., 1993). There is also anecdotal evidence to suggest that the turnover of staff in charities generally and adoption societies in particular is less than in other sectors. With a general shortage of sufficiently skilled and trained professionals in adoption, it will be increasingly necessary to look at ways of making use of this available expertise before much of it disappears through the natural process of retirement. Specialist workers who regularly make placements clearly have more experience as to what works and doesn't work in family placement. This specialism could be shared by secondments of local authority workers to voluntary agencies providing them with an opportunity to explore adoption from a different perspective. Joint training, adoption panel member exchanges, joint recruitment campaigns and shared preparation groups for adopters are all useful ways for the two sectors to work more closely together.

Voluntary adoption agencies are not organisational islands but operate within a broader environment in which the voluntary/statutory relationships are key 'in an era where partnership is increasingly becoming the working pattern for public authorities' (Department of Environment, Transport and the Regions, 2000). In adoption, it may be argued that partnership is intrinsically unequal in the sense that voluntary agencies only have access to children available for adoption through local authorities except in the case of a small minority of infant placements. Nevertheless, in 1999, 29 voluntary agencies placed 25 per cent of those looked-after children who were placed for adoption.

At the moment, voluntary agencies are in great demand for their families as Quality Protects challenges local authorities with placement targets. This demand is likely to continue in the next few years as government policy aims to increase by 40 per cent the number of looked-after children adopted by 2004–5. However, the government's adoption review team (Performance and Innovation Unit, 2000) was right to reject the rather fanciful notion of removing adoption responsibilities from local authorities. Expansion of mainstream adoption work into the voluntary sector could well be counter-productive. Even if the agencies had the capacity to respond to larger numbers and absorb additional work, the reality of voluntary sector response to statutory agendas is complex. Such a development might well involve them in a distortion of mission, a compromise of values or an undermining of the ethos and identity of their working practices. There is evidence to highlight the unequal nature of voluntary/statutory partnerships which are hastily assembled to implement government initiatives as well as the continuing importance of less formalised relationships between the sectors despite the prevailing contract culture (Scott *et al.*, 2000).

Partnership is inevitably linked to issues about funding. At present, all voluntary adoption agencies subsidise their adoption work to a greater or lesser extent through charitable income. This added value may be argued as a legitimate use of resources particularly since much of it goes on post-adoption work for which there is currently no statutory funding. The Consortium of Voluntary Adoption Agencies calculated this contribution from their 29 members at over £2.5 million per annum in 1999.

There are excellent examples of partnership in the adoption world. One such, which transcends the traditional relationships between voluntary and statutory agencies, is Adoption – A Quality Option Project. This initiative, funded by the Department of Health, enabled the Catholic Children's Society (Nottingham), a small agency with a wealth of experience and resources in adoption, to develop a two-year partnership with a number of local authorities. Participating authorities were able to reflect on the complex demands adoption places on local councils, concentrate on some of the structural problems which affect time scales and planning for children and consider the impact of this interplay on other systems concerned in the adoption process. Effective systems for tracking children through the care system were devised thus better informing their assessment for adoption placements. The same organisation has earlier, through their Project 16–18: Adoption in my Life, disseminated research findings of national importance and made available teaching resources to a wide audience about the needs of young people in adoption. Research information included direct evidence from young people via an interactive website. This data suggested that young people who feel they have a lot of background information are more positive about being adopted; that access to the internet and telephone helplines addressed young people's need to find information quickly and with relative anonymity; that families were seen as the most helpful source of information about adoption but it was nevertheless not an easy subject for young people to raise.

Voluntary adoption agencies have an important role in developing and monitoring new initiatives. An excellent example of this is the new concurrent planning project, developed by Coram Family's adoption service and others, which aims to reduce the length of time that very young children wait in the care of local authorities before decisions are made about their future (see Gray, Chapter 3). The pilot scheme provides looked-after children with a permanent alternative family from the outset. The idea is that this family will adopt the child if returning to the birth family proves impossible.

The nature of voluntary adoption societies as charities gives them access to different sources of funding from government, trusts and corporate donors for innovative developmental work. With it comes the freedom to take risks and the ability to focus very closely on specific areas of work such as post-adoption, direct work with birth families, therapeutic work with children, sibling placements or organised groups for adopted adolescents. Some voluntary adoption societies are particularly skilled in recruiting families from minority ethnic communities and it has been suggested that, given the number of 'waiting' children, more local authorities should be encouraged to refer black children to the voluntary sector (Ivaldi, 2000).

Voluntary sector independence is not, however, just about sources of income. It is also about choice. Choices in adoption apply not just to adopters but also to children and their birth families. Voluntary adoption agencies can act as a mediator or buffer between the State and the individual, between private responsibilities and public responses. The nature of an independent provider can be an invaluable aid when local authorities have to address the fundamental dilemma which occurs when child protection separates the child's best interest from the needs of the parents. Independent, experienced adoption workers can assist local authorities identify children for whom permanent placement would be appropriate. The same experience might also be useful in resisting pressure for adoption where this is not appropriate. External stimulus can help ensure timely progress for children whatever the plan. The Family Rights Group and others have consistently cautioned against adoption being viewed as a panacea and less priority being given to keeping families together. In fact, adoption skills require an appreciation of the effects of this primary bond and the value of family, race, culture and religion in the life of the child. It may therefore also be very appropriate for local authorities to offer a more independent service to birth parents whose children are going through care proceedings and may be in dispute with the social services department. Much creative work has been undertaken by voluntary agencies with birth parents in difficult circumstances and post-adoption centres have run groups for birth parents and relatives. Practice guidelines on intermediary services for birth relatives (Department of Health, 2000) were developed by the Children's Society drawing on their own large-scale research study (see Howe and Feast, 2000 and Chapter 3).

Voluntary organisations also fulfil a key role in providing information and resources to the general public about adoption and the wider needs of children. Adoption UK (the former Parent to Parent Information Services on Adoption), NORCAP and the Adoption Forum are all examples of organisations whose links with local communities can enhance self-help, mutual aid resources and networks. Voluntary sector helplines like Talk Adoption, because of their neutrality and independence, provide important routes into both statutory and voluntary services for adopted adults, young people, birth parents and adopters. This work can be undertaken without the distraction of heavy bombardment rates affecting social services departments or the spread of other children's priority services like child protection or political intervention. The luxury of this position cannot be overstated. It enables voluntary agencies to promote public debate from a different viewpoint within the wider childcare world. Although children are now firmly placed on the political agenda, the modernisation programme and subsequent overload in planning and service delivery places local authorities under enormous pressure. Yet, as a former social services director wrote: 'When everything is a priority, nothing is: the message for ministers and senior managers alike is to keep an eye on the big picture – the overall direction of change – and not get sucked into micro-management' (Bamford, 2000). This consideration applies equally in the field of adoption where the level of challenge presented by some of the most deeply troubled children is huge and overrides agency or sector sensibilities. It demands a consistent multi-agency service for children and families which far surpasses what is currently on offer individually from either sector, statutory or voluntary.

References

Association of British Fostering and Adoption Agencies (1976), Voluntary agencies in peril (editorial), *Adoption and Fostering*, 3.

Bamford, T. (2000), An eye on the big picture, *Guardian*, 23 August 2000.

Billis, D. and Harris, M. (eds) (1996), *Voluntary agencies: challenges of organisation and management*, London, Macmillan.

Department of Health (2000), *Intermediary services for birth relatives*, London, Department of Health.

Department of the Environment, Transport and the Regions (2000), *Local compact guidelines*, London, Department of the Environment, Transport and the Regions.

Howe, D. and Feast, J. (2000), *Adoption, Search and Reunion*, London, Children's Society.

Howe, D., Sawbridge, P. and Hining, D. (1992), *Half a million women*, Harmondsworth, Penguin Books.

Ivaldi, G. (2000), *Children and families in the voluntary sector*, London, British Agencies for Adoption and Fostering.

Lowe, N., Murch, M., Borowski, M., Copner, R. and Griew, R. (1993), *Pathways to adoption*, Research Project, HMSO, in R. Parker (ed.) (1999), *Adoption now: messages from research*, Chichester, John Wiley & Sons.

Performance and Innovation Unit (2000), *Review on adoption: Issues for Consultation*, London, The Cabinet Office.

Rowe, J. (1996), *Parents, children and adoption*, London, Routledge.

Scott, D., Alcock, P., Russell, L. and Macmillan, R. (2000), *Moving pictures: realities of voluntary action*, Bristol, The Policy Press.

Wigmore, B. (1996), The sins of the fathers, *New Statesman*, 4 October 1996.

30

ADOPTION IN NEW ZEALAND

An international perspective

Jill Goldson

The first country in the British Empire to legalise adoption in 1881, New Zealand continues seriously to review adoption policy at the beginning of the new century. As in other countries, social changes have impacted on adoption, for example, state financial support for single parents, access to abortion, and progress in reproductive technology. Within this context of change, New Zealand has been leading the way as a country practising and succeeding in open adoption.

This current interpretation of the Adoption Act 1955 is a far cry from the deep secrecy that characterised the process in the middle of the last century. Back then, primary consideration was given to the perceived need to protect the involved parties from the respective stigmas of illegitimacy and infertility. Young pregnant women were sent to the country to live out their pregnancy and delivery in secret whilst prospective adoptive mothers are known to have simulated pregnancy in the months before adoption by means of the strategic positioning of a pillow.

The assumption that a single mother would want to make a fresh start, without her baby and free of stigma, was fuelled by theorists such as John Bowlby whose work on attachment theory and its implications for early bonding reinforced the 'clean break' approach. Newborn infants were at a premium in contrast to the years between 1890 and 1930 when 'children of "useful" years' were seen to be less of an economic liability than small babies (Tennant, 1985). In fact, prior to World War II, many mothers did not give up their babies for adoption; should she be unable to care for her infant, institutional care often resulted.

After the war the New Zealand government became concerned about the cost to the state of keeping children in institutions and spoke emotively about the moral decline of society. Social values espoused the notion of a stable childhood only being possible in a nuclear family. Child welfare services became actively involved in promoting the desirability of placing children with families on a permanent basis by means of legal, closed adoption. The birth family was discounted as being of no real importance to the child and birth mothers were often told that they were not allowed to attempt to find their child. Adoption Regulations in 1959 allowed the identities of the adoptive parents to be kept secret by identifying them only with a number if they so wished. 'Closed stranger adoption can now be seen for what it was – a social experiment with unknown and uninvestigated outcomes conducted on a massive scale' (Else, 1991).

Running parallel to adoption legislation, and predating it by hundreds of years, is the Maori customary practice of adoption called whangai. This practice, still occurring today, involves none of the secrecy that has surrounded pakeha (European) practice. The Maori child is placed in the wider family and not only knows his birth parents but usually has contact with them. The child remains connected within his cultural context and the placement serves to strengthen relations with the extended family or tribe. The legal transfer and severing of a child's heritage is foreign to Maori. Although varying degrees of recognition have been afforded these customary placements in New Zealand, the current legislation (the Adoption Act 1955) confirms that whangai since 1909 has only limited legal effect. The imposition of a monocultural social policy, in the centre of the customary adoption triangle, is seen by its critics as both an imposition and as oppressive.

These negative effects were highlighted after the trend in the early 1960s for Maori children to be adopted into white families. Such children were cut off from family ties completely and not able to trace their biological roots until the passing of the Adult Information Act in 1985. It is very probable that such policy had a major impact on the mental health of Maori adoptees.

Maori have continued to use whangai placement as a means of caring for children and at present there appears to be only limited support for specific legal recognition of whangai. A more favoured approach appears to be that of an underlying philosophical base to adoption law which incorporates Maori values into its legislation. These values would need to be applied according to the tikanga (protocol) supporting each circumstance.

Meanwhile, key changes were taking place in the sociology of family life; The Status of Children Act 1969, removed discrimination from illegitimacy, financial state benefits supported single mothers and abortion became more accessible, as did effective contraception. The women's movement set up fundamental challenges to the status quo and the ideology of the family began to shift. This coincided with a rise in popularity for theories such as existentialism which promoted freedom of choice and superceded a prior preoccupation with psychoanalytic theories. The work of Erik Erikson on identity formation highlighted the importance of knowing one's roots.

The Adult Information Act catalysed the push towards the trend to open adoption practice in New Zealand. This act came about after a long campaign starting in the 1970s by pressure groups such as Jigsaw and allowed the adopted person 20 years and over the right to apply for a copy of their original birth certificate along with other identifying information about their birth parent. Access to information is only blocked if there is a veto in place which prevents the release of identifying information. Such vetoes last for 10 years but can be cancelled or renewed at any time.

If no veto has been placed by the birth parents, the birth certificate is sent to a counsellor chosen by the adopted person. The certificate is then released in a mandatory interview, leaving the way clear for a search and contact to be made at the adoptee's own pace. Similarly, the birth parent or parents seeking the release of their adopted child's name can make application under this act and if no veto exists, a social worker from the specialist adoptions unit in the statutory child, youth and family department, will endeavour to find the adopted person and seek their permission for identifying information to be released. Birth parents are not required to attend a mandatory interview.

A six-month moratorium is observed before the release of identifying information in order to give the people concerned the opportunity to consider placing a veto and counselling is made available to anyone involved in this process.

The passing of this law signified a major change in the view that birth mothers needed to make a fresh start. Implicit in this is the acknowledgment that society has a responsibility to adopted people and their birth parents to provide information which can restore peace of mind and address unresolved issues. The system of vetoes has declined significantly in the last 10 years, a trend likely to continue.

Access to identifying information by others, such as grandparents, adopted parents and siblings are still excluded under the Act. However, the original Adoption Act 1955 has a section for release of information under special circumstances.

Consideration is currently being given in proposals (Law Commission, 2000) which would allow a three-year period after which no more new vetoes could be placed. Although the current system of vetoes denies access to the information on the birth register, it does not prevent people affected by adoption from seeking further information in registers held in public libraries.

Over the past two decades there has been a dramatic change in adoption practice in New Zealand. The country has been described as 'leading the world in practising, and succeeding at, open adoption arrangements' (Law Commission, 2000). Most adoptions now involve some degree of contact from the very beginning of the adoption arrangement. The country's specialist adoption unit provides birth parents with the opportunity to make an input in the selection of adoptive parents by giving them personal profiles made up by the adoptive applicants and thus giving them an overview of their lifestyle, values and aspirations. This process simultaneously gives the prospective adoptive parents the potential for a greater sense of entitlement to parent someone else's child. A non-binding contract is then signed at the adoption creating an individual and flexible arrangement setting out the contact that will be kept.

A downward trend in adoptions can be observed: 90 per cent of stranger adoptions are open adoptions (that is, some contact agreed). The proportion of stranger to non-stranger adoptions has changed dramatically from the 1960s on. This trend seems set to continue: in 1993–4 there were 683 total adoptions, 183 of which were stranger adoptions, and in 2000–1 the numbers were 382 total adoptions and 78 stranger adoptions, according to figures from the Adoption Information Services Unit of Child Youth and Family in 2002.

Inter-country adoptions have emerged as an option much later in New Zealand than in other countries. Up until 1988, most inter-country adoptions were relative adoptions from Western Samoa. The decline in local adoptions has led to a growth of interest in inter country adoptions and New Zealand is a signatory to the Hague Convention, which is a detailed international regulatory framework.

Although open adoption is widely practised in New Zealand, it is not tacitly recognised in law and although the Adult Information Act has gone a long way towards addressing the issues of secrecy, philosophically the practice is at odds with the 47-year-old Act. Much considered thought is currently being given to the future and form of adoption in New Zealand. Whilst the concept of adoption is generally accepted as serving an important purpose, those who are currently researching the issues are committed to a wide range of reforms. Proposed reforms have been discussed and tabled in a Law Commission document inquiring into adoption. The options were published in 2000.

There is fundamental agreement that the principle of the interests of the child being paramount (which informs the Child Youth and Family Act in this country as well as the Guardianship Act) must continue to inform adoption legislation. In this respect, it has been suggested that one of the key areas relating to the child's best interests is the evaluation of whether alternatives to adoption would better suit that child.

To this end, serious consideration was given to the concept of a proposed new act called the Care of Children Act. This act would incorporate adoption, child protection and guardianship legislation thus creating a spectrum of care. Arrangements for the temporary care of children would sit at one end of the spectrum. At the other end, a reformulated concept of adoption would be defined. Hence, disparate pieces of legislation would be brought together within a coherent continuum characterised by an ease of movement between the options. A key principle embedded in this proposal is that children are provided with a full range of legal options for permanent placements, whether adoptive or otherwise. Caregivers for the child would be afforded legal rights and responsibilities for the child under the proposed legislation.

This vision condemns the provision in the Adoption Act which deems an adopted child to be born of adoptive parents as both anachronistic and repugnant, distorting reality and setting up a legal fiction. It is argued that parental responsibility can be transferred in law from the birth parents to the caregivers or adoptive parents but simultaneously a birth family still exists and may have a role in a child's life. This transparent process would be reflected in a parenting plan where issues arising in open adoption would be addressed. It is envisaged that support services such as mediation and counselling would be readily available to the parties to expedite arrangements made in the parenting plan.

Also recommended is the provision of two birth certificates upon registration of an adoption order: a post-adoption certificate which only shows the adoptive parents, and a full birth certificate that lists all the details of the person's birth and subsequent adoption. Access as of right would be restricted to the persons named on the certificate. Anyone else seeking access would need to establish proper personal interest through the Family Court or have permission from the adopted person.

Unfortunately, these proposed reforms have not been taken up and there is no consensus currently between the two major political parties on the subject. The arena for debate and discussion, however, has been firmly established.

Social legislation needs to resonate with changing mores. When it lags behind the values and expectations of new generations, unanticipated yet deep conflict can arise. Adoption law remains important as an option amongst a range of options for the future care of a child whose parents can no longer fulfil that task. The viability of the concept of adoption in New Zealand depends on the ability of legislators to capture and codify the changing needs of families and their children.

References

Else, A. (1991), *Closed stranger adoption*, Wellington, Bridget Williams Books.

Law Commission (2000), Report 65, *Adoption and its alternatives: a different approach and a new framework.*

Tennant, M. (1985), Maternity and morality: homes for single mothers 1890–1930, *Women's Studies Journal,* 2(1), 28.

31

ADOPTION IS ABOUT PEOPLE

Learning the lessons of experience

John Simmonds

Adoption has undergone more change in recent times than for a quarter of a century. It has been one of those rare times when the chance presents itself to mark a generation. This change has ushered in a new legal framework, adoption standards, practice guidance, an adoption register, an adoption and permanency council, a task force and targets and indicators. From a sleepy and marginalised issue in social work and social policy, adoption is now centre stage. With all the energy, drive and resources that these new developments command, it is vital that we do not see this as just a new beginning but that we can learn from history and experience and not repeat past mistakes.

One of the complex issues that the theme of learning from experience must address is how to incorporate the experience of those people who have been personally touched by adoption. This itself is not a new theme as consumer views, participation and involvement in public services have become an important influence in the planning and delivery of those services. More specifically there has been the gradual development of services in the statutory, voluntary and self help sectors that have given people affected by adoption an opportunity to explore, express and validate their own experiences and views in an area where secrecy, misunderstanding and confusion have been all too common.

Indeed, it is absolutely critical that all these developments actually directly benefit those people most affected by them. The risk, of course, is that the reputation of politicians or government or the needs of bureaucracies, agencies or adoption professionals will come to dominate the agenda for change. Power and power relations are instrumental in bringing about change but history often tells us that such efforts are sometimes not good in delivering the benefits to consumers of the change they actually bring about.

One of the great difficulties with the principal of ensuring that services are of direct benefit to service users in adoption is the nature of the subject itself.

While there are tangible issues that can be measured like the time taken to approve adopters or the time it takes to find placements for children, or the number of children placed for adoption, much adoption experience inhabits a rather different world. Adoption is a world infused with a complex set of life-long relationships, with emotion as the currency and the capacity to create meaningful lives the goal. Hard and fast rules, certainty and particularly the current fashionable language of political and organisational change with its focus on achievement, making a difference, targets and performance outcomes do not sit easily in this world. Adoption inhabits more of an intermediate world where hope and despair, the past, present and future both coexist and collide. There is the ever-present potential for conflict and the certainty of loss. A child's need and hope for a permanent family through adoption and all that that might mean throughout his or her life will collide with, but need to co-exist with the loss of life with the birth family. A new beginning for one person in adoption invariably means loss for others. For the adoptive parents, it will mean the fulfilment of their wish for a child but the probable loss of the birth child for which they hoped, where infertility is a motivating factor. For the birth parents, it means the loss of their birth child but a new opportunity for that child or themselves to build a different life elsewhere.

And the list of losses and gains can go on and on, for different people in different relationships to the adoption, all with their own perspectives on what the event might mean for them. But even then this is never straightforward as these experiences are never locked into a certainty for all time. Loss, conflict, uncertainty, guilt, regret and pain, as well as hope, excitement, joy and exhilaration – indeed a wide range of powerful and sometimes disturbing feelings – weave their way throughout adoption affecting different people in different ways at different times and rarely with the certainty of knowing that how we feel today is how we will feel tomorrow. My own experiences as an adoptive father for 21 years still leave me open to feelings that I had never anticipated or others that are the opposite of what I have felt at other times in my life.

But for all the fluidity of actual experience, from whoever's experience and perspective one looks at it, the questions that frequently arise are – was this a good thing that happened? Was this a good thing that you did? Has it worked out or has it been a failure? These are some of the demanding and difficult questions faced by many adoption agencies as they struggle, secretly or openly, to gain a respectable place in politically sensitive national league tables. Have they done enough, have they done it right and can they prove it? They are also the demanding and difficult questions faced by birth parents, adopted children and adults and adoptive parents as they struggle, secretly or openly, to make sense of their own circumstances and their own decisions – have they done enough, have they done it right and can they justify it?

In this intermediate world where experiences both collide and coexist, individuals are faced with constructing meaning out of a reality that is made up of different emotions at different times and with different intensities. Could I have tried harder? If only I had done this or if I hadn't done or said that. Is my loss, their gain or is my gain their loss? If they weren't like that or if I was this kind of person or it hadn't happened in quite that kind of way. These are the kinds of questions one asks oneself or the statements which arise. Facing past regrets, doubts, wishes and hopes or current realities, future plans or uncertainties without being overwhelmed by confusion and anxiety or anaesthetising oneself to their impact are critical. Facing and relating to this complex intermediate world and creating meaning out of its many different faces is the challenge of adoption.

With the complexity of these questions and issues, it is not surprising that people use defences to stop themselves being overwhelmed. Ideology and rigidity of both thought and organisational systems often seem to pervade adoption. They may not be defensive in their intention but can be defensive in their outcome by providing individuals and organisations with a powerful sense of security and knowing where they stand.

The history of adoption has all too often been marked by these defences as individuals and agencies struggle to find ways of making sense out of experience. What is quite striking about this history is the extent to which it has resulted in territorial and boundary disputes that are characterised by all the emotions of larger scale territorial and boundary disputes – mistrust, hostility, betrayal, closed borders or open warfare. There are so many things which create the risk of conflicts and disputes, the potential or actual ferocity of which, make defensive and ideological positions either necessary or attractive – the absolute and rigid secrecy that has, in the past, surrounded the shame and guilt of an unplanned or unwanted child; the secrecy or lies that have been used to manage the anxiety of telling a child that they are adopted or giving them access to birth information; the fierce and damaging conflict over the unacceptability or advantages of transracial placements or overseas adoption; the rage and despair at that small group of birth parents who so damage or neglect their birth children that alternative family care becomes a necessity; or the rage and despair of birth parents or birth families whose rights and responsibilities for, or interest in their children have been permanently terminated by state intervention. This is a matter of having to seem to be for or against and deciding which.

Adoption cannot be thought of as an anaesthetic to the pain of the past, present or future. It cannot be thought of as a defence against infertility, a defence against the problems of the care system, a defence against thoughts and feelings, or a defence against about what has happened even if we wish it hadn't. It is a living thing that moves and changes and struggles to grow. It may provide solutions to complex issues, but it cannot be thought of as resolving a problem that exists at one moment in time for the rest of time.

Adoption is a living thing that requires real people to engage in real issues. It requires commitment, determination, support and open communication. It needs a language and a way of relating that is marked by creativity, playfulness, sensitivity and fluidity of thinking.

These issues mark some of the struggles parents have to confront in both understanding and creating the conditions which promote and facilitate the healthy development of children. Children need to be exposed to experiences and knowledge about their history and circumstances in a way that makes sense relative to the stage they have reached in their development. Present them with too much and they will not understand or will be overwhelmed. Present them with too little and they will be starved of the raw material that stimulates and enables growth.

But what is too much and what too little? When is the right time to talk about the complexities of sex or drugs or expose children to the inevitability of adult conflict or violence or the idea of dangerous people? How do you explain the circumstances of birth parents in a sensitive and sensible way without creating untruths or giving misleading information? How do you explain that you gave up your child for adoption or had one removed by social workers and the courts and your wishes in the matter overruled? How do you explain that your first thought every morning as you wake up is for that child when you have a new family who needs you? How do you explain to your adoptive parents that you are desperate to make contact with your birth parents when you fear that they will feel betrayed? Where, with any of these and many, many more do you give meaning to these experiences, make your stand and act? And can you do so in a way that is marked by creative, playful, sensitive and fluid thinking rather than thinking that is marked by an ideological position and rigidity of thought?

This is one of the great challenges for the new framework and system of adoption that will emerge from contemporary changes. At its best, what is sought from the change is driven by the desire to create stability and a greater sense of permanence for children who need secure and loving families. There are too many children living in damaging circumstances where the love, commitment, and determination of parents are absent. These situations invite a real sense of outrage and concern and a demand that something be done – and of course that is right. They are also an invitation to find somebody or something to blame. They demand a solution that rescues children and us from unacceptable situations. And the solution should leave us satisfied in the knowledge that we have succeeded or, at least, can demonstrate that we have succeeded. Unfortunately, this is precisely the kind of scenario that the public services are confronted with again and again: unacceptable situations that invite outrage, then blame, then defensive solutions that appear to demonstrate that we have moved things on. It is an issue for health services, transport services, social services and, indeed, it can be for adoption. But is this really learning the lessons of history? Is this really listening to what people have to tell us about their experiences, wishes and needs, about the complexity of their lives, the losses and gains, the challenges and disappointments, the frustration and achievements?

We need to find solutions but they do not come without space for listening, understanding, tolerance and sensitivity. These are the values that might really help us to think and in the in the end know that we have made a difference to people in a way that counts.

INDEX